Contents

Handbook of Breast Cancer Risk-Assessment

Evidence-Based Guidelines for Evaluation, Prevention, Counseling, and Treatment

Victor G. Vogel, MD, MHS
Therese Bevers, MD

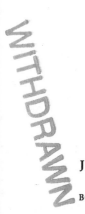

JONES AND BARTLETT PUBLISHERS
Sudbury, Massachusetts
BOSTON   TORONTO   LONDON   SINGAPORE

World Headquarters

Jones and Bartlett
Publishers
40 Tall Pine Drive
Sudbury, MA 01776
978-443-5000
info@jbpub.com
www.jbpub.com

Jones and Bartlett
Publishers Canada
2406 Nikanna Road
Mississauga,
ON L5C 2W6
CANADA

Jones and Bartlett
Publishers International
Barb House, Barb Mews
London W6 7PA
UK

Library of Congress Cataloging-in-Publication Data
Handbook of breast cancer risk-assessment : evidence-based guidelines for evalua-
tion, prevention, counseling, and treatment / edited by Victor G. Vogel, Therese
Bevers.
    p. ; cm.
Includes bibliographical references and index.
ISBN 0-7637-1860-2 (alk. paper)
    1. Breast--Cancer--Risk factors--Handbooks, manuals, etc. 2. Breast--Cancer--
Patients--Counseling of--Handbooks, manuals, etc. 3. Health risk assessment--
Handbooks, manuals, etc. 4. Evidence-based medicine--Handbooks, manuals, etc.
    [DNLM: 1. Breast Neoplasms--prevention & control--Handbooks. 2. Evidence-Based
Medicine--Handbooks. 3. Genetic Counseling--Handbooks. 4. Risk Assessment--
Handbooks. WP 39 H2335 2003] I. Vogel, Victor G. II. Bevers, Therese.
RC280.B8 H359 2003
616.99'449--dc21

                                                                            2002014830

Production Credits
Executive Publisher: Christopher Davis
Production Manager: Amy Rose
Associate Editor: Karen Zuck
Associate Production Editor: Karen C. Ferreira
Production Assistant: Jenny McIsaac
Senior Marketing Manager: Alisha Weisman
Manufacturing Buyer: Amy Bacus
Text and Cover Design: Anne Spencer
Composition: Carlisle Publishers Services
Printing and Binding: Malloy Lithographing
Cover Printing: Malloy Lithographing

Printed in the United States of America
07 06 05 04 03   10 9 8 7 6 5 4 3 2 1

With the identification of breast cancer susceptibility genes and a computerized breast cancer risk assessment tool now available for use in the clinical setting, evaluation of a woman's risk of breast cancer has revolutionized the approach to the primary and secondary prevention of breast cancer. In the past decade, the paradigm has shifted from screening recommendations standardized by age to risk reduction and screening guidelines that are based on personalized risk assessment.

Only through identification of increased risk of developing breast cancer can we determine if breast cancer screening should be instituted earlier or whether risk reduction strategies should be considered. A thorough understanding of breast cancer risk and how risks balance against benefits is required to guide a woman and her physician in the decisions to be made. Significant experience has accumulated during the past decade that now guides recommendations for establishing and operating specialized clinics devoted to evaluation and management of women who are at increased risk for breast cancer.

Lifestyle modification can be suggested as a healthy and prudent maneuver for all women, whether they are at average or increased risk. Its benefit in reducing breast cancer risk, however, remains uncertain. Prophylactic surgical strategies (mastectomy and oophorectomy) confer significant reduction of breast cancer risk, but are reserved primarily for those with genetic predisposition because the physiological and psychological consequences can be significant. A thorough knowledge of genetic counseling and testing is also required to manage risk adequately and appropriately. With the demonstration that tamoxifen can reduce breast cancer risk by almost one-half, chemoprevention is emerging as the primary intervention strategy for most women at increased risk of the disease. Tamoxifen carries with it, though, the possibility of rare but significant harm, and counseling is imperative so that a woman understands the potential risks and benefits of therapy and makes an informed decision about the management of her risk.

The information in this manual will equip the healthcare provider with the tools needed to assess a woman's risk of developing breast cancer and to advise her about the appropriate options available to reduce her risk.

Victor G. Vogel, MD, MHS

Therese Bevers, MD

chapter 1

Epidemiology of Breast Cancer

Victor G. Vogel, MD, MHS, FACP
Professor of Medicine and Epidemiology
Director, Magee/University of Pittsburgh Cancer Institute
Breast Program, Magee-Womens Hospital
Pittsburgh, PA

I.   Factors That Increase Risk of Breast Cancer (Table 1.1)

   A. While age-adjusted incidence of breast cancer has risen 1 to 2% per year over the past 50 years, mortality from breast cancer began to fall in North America and Western Europe in the mid-1990s.[1]

   B. Risk factors identify women who require special management and increase our understanding of the biological processes that lead to breast cancer.[2–7]

   C. Risk is a relative term derived by comparing the incidence of a disease in a group having a particular risk factor or trait with the incidence of the same disease in a comparison group of individuals who do not carry the risk factor but who are in every other way the same.

      1. Risk can be expressed as the odds ratio (the ratio of the odds of having the disease in those with the trait of interest compared with the odds of having the disease in those without the trait).

      2. Risk can also be expressed as the ratio of the incidence of the disease in those with the trait divided by the incidence of the disease in those without the trait. This is the relative

TABLE 1.1	Risk Factors for Breast Cancer and Their Relative Risks		
Risk Factor*	Comparison Category	Risk Category	Relative Risk
Age at menarche	16 years	Younger than 12 years	1.3
Age at menopause	45 to 54 years	After 55 years	1.5
Age when first child born alive	Before 20 years	Nulliparous or older than 30 years	1.9
Benign breast disease	No biopsy or fine needle aspiration	Any benign disease	1.5
		Proliferative disease	2.0
		Atypical hyperplasia	4.0
Family history of breast cancer	No first-degree relative affected	Mother affected	1.7
		Two first-degree relatives affected	5.0
Obesity	10th percentile	90th percentile	1.2
Alcohol use	Nondrinker	Moderate drinker	1.7
Estrogen replacement therapy	Never used	Current use ≥ 3 years	1.5

Source: Harris JR, Lippman ME, Veronesi U, Willett W. Breast cancer. *N Engl J Med.* 1992;327:319–328.

Relative risks represent median values reported in the published literature.

risk, that is, the level of increased risk of developing the disease associated with the risk factor.

3. The relationship between a risk factor and the proportion of cases of a disease that it may cause is known as the attributable risk.

4. Calculation of the attributable risk requires only that we know the prevalence of a particular risk factor in the population of interest and the relative risk associated with that risk factor.

D. Age

1. The most important single risk factor is age.

2. The annual incidence of breast cancer in the United States among women 80 to 85 years of age is 15 times higher than the incidence of breast cancer among women 30 to 35 years of age.[8]

   a. 412 cases per 100,000 women per year at age 80

   b. 27.9 cases per 100,000 women per year at age 30

3. It is not known if these observed differences are explained by the accumulation of a number of events that occur throughout a woman's lifetime or by a single event that is triggered with greater frequency in older as compared with younger women.

E. Race and ethnicity modify the effect of age on the risk of breast cancer.

1. African-American women younger than 50 years have a higher age-specific incidence of breast cancer than their white American women counterparts, but older African-American women have a lower age-specific incidence than older white American women.

2. Breast cancer incidence among Hispanic women living in North America is only 40 to 50% as great as the incidence among non-Hispanic white women.

3. Asian women born in Asia have an extremely low lifetime risk of breast cancer, but their daughters born in North America have the same lifetime risk of breast cancer as white American women.

4. No explanation, including dietary factors, yet accounts for these observed differences in breast cancer incidence.

F. Gynecological events

1. Most breast cancer risk factors relate to gynecological or endocrinological events that occur in a woman's lifetime.[9]

2. Age at menarche is related to a woman's chance of developing breast cancer:

   a. Compared with women who experience menarche at age 16, girls who experience menarche 2 to 5 years earlier have a 10 to 30% greater risk of developing breast cancer later in life.

3. Age at menopause

   a. The average age at menopause in the United States is slightly older than 51 years.

   b. Compared to women who experience menopause between the ages of 45 and 55 years as the referent group, women who experience menopause at age 55 or older have a 50% higher risk of subsequently developing breast cancer.

   c. Women who cease menstruating at age 45 or younger have a 30% lower risk of subsequently developing breast cancer.
   d. One way of expressing the risk of breast cancer in relation to gynecological events is to count the number of ovulatory menstrual cycles that a woman experiences in her lifetime.

4. *Early menarche and late menopause lead to an increased total lifetime number of menstrual cycles and a corresponding 30 to 50% increase in breast cancer risk.*

5. *Late menarche and early menopause lead to a reduction in breast cancer risk of similar magnitude.*

6. *Oophorectomy before the age of menopause (especially before the age of 40) lowers the risk of breast cancer by approximately two-thirds.*

G. Circulating estrogen levels

   1. *In adult women, the predominant circulating estrogen is estradiol.*
      a. Most estradiol is bound to sex hormone binding globulin (SHBG).
      b. A smaller proportion of estradiol is bound to albumin.

   2. *Between menarche and menopause, a woman is exposed to higher static levels of circulating estradiol (bound to either SHBG or albumin, as well as freely circulating).*

   3. *In meta-analyses, plasma estradiol levels are 15 to 25% higher in breast cancer cases compared with control subjects.*

   4. *Circulating levels of DHEA, prolactin, and IGF-I are associated with an increased risk of breast cancer with differing effects among premenopausal and postmenopausal women.*[10,11]

H. Cell proliferation is low during the follicular phase of the menstrual cycle and does not increase with the preovulatory peak in estradiol.

   1. *Following ovulation, progesterone stimulates cell proliferation to three times the follicular rates.*

   2. *If fertilization and pregnancy do not occur, progesterone levels fall, breast cell division decreases, and apoptosis follows.*

   3. *During pregnancy, circulating levels of both estrogen and progesterone remain elevated.*

   4. *Progesterone is a potent mitogen to breast cells, possibly making them more susceptible to the effects of breast carcinogens or promoting substances.*

   5. *During the second half of pregnancy, cell differentiation occurs in the breast, and proliferation decreases.*

I. Pregnancy at a young age, especially before the age of 20, markedly reduces the incidence of subsequent breast cancer.

   1. *Both nulliparity and age older than 30 years at first live birth are associated with nearly a doubling of the risk of subsequent breast cancer.*

   2. *Pregnancies not ending in the birth of a viable fetus do not confer reduction in the risk of breast cancer.*

   3. *Spontaneous abortion does not increase the relative risk of breast cancer among parous women, while induced abortion*

may increase the risk of breast cancer in nulliparous women (RR = 1.3, 95% CI = 0.9–1.9).

4. *There are no data from women that provide a histological explanation for the protection from breast cancer brought about by early pregnancy.*

5. *An increased number of lifetime ovulatory menstrual cycles increases the risk of breast cancer. This can occur with early age at menarche, late age at menopause, and/or few or no full-term pregnancies.*

6. *Lactation for two or more years decreases the lifetime risk of breast cancer by at least 50%, but this may be confined only to women with increased parity.*

7. *The risk of breast cancer increases by approximately 3% per year of delayed menopause (average age at menopause in North America is approximately 51 years).*

8. *The risk of breast cancer associated with the use of oral contraceptives returns to baseline ten years after use of OCPs is discontinued (data from 50 published studies).*

J. Benign breast disease

1. *Some studies show a correlation between risk factors for breast cancer and those for benign breast disease.*

2. *Benign disease is not more common in women with other risk factors for breast cancer such as a family history of the disease.*[12]

3. *Fewer than 20% of women in North America have undergone a biopsy for benign breast disease by age 50.*[13]

4. *Benign breast disease that results in biopsy increases the risk of subsequently developing breast cancer.*

5. *The risk of breast cancer after undergoing biopsy for benign breast disease is not uniform. The subsequent risk is greater in premenopausal than in postmenopausal women who have a breast biopsy.*[2]

   a. Biopsy before the age of 50 to 55 years may be associated with a fivefold to sixfold increase in the risk of breast cancer.

   b. Biopsy at older ages is associated with only half this risk.

6. *An accepted classification schema divides benign disease into proliferative and nonproliferative categories.*[14,15]

   a. The important subclassifications of proliferative disease are listed in Table 1.2 with their associated relative risks.

   b. Proliferative disease accounts for between one-fourth and one-third of all biopsies for benign disease.

   c. Five to 10% of proliferative lesions show cellular atypia, the histologic change associated with the highest risk of subsequent breast cancer.

   d. Atypical features are similar to some found in carcinoma *in situ.*

   e. A family history of breast cancer in first-degree relatives has an additive effect on the subsequent risk of breast cancer in women with atypia.

   f. Increasing use of mammographic screening has led to increased identification of women with proliferative lesions of the breast.

TABLE 1.2	Classification of Benign Breast Disease and the Risk for Subsequent Development of Breast Cancer		
		Relative Risk for Breast Cancer	
Benign Lesion	Description	With Family History	No Family History
Proliferative disease without atypia		2.4–2.7	1.7–1.9
Moderate and florid ductal hyperplasia of the usual type	Most common type of hyperplasia; cells do not have the cytologic appearance of lobular or apocrinelike lesions; florid lesions have a proliferation of cells that fill more than 70% of the involved space		
Additional lesions	Intraductal papilloma, radial scar, sclerosing adenosis, apocrine metaplasia		
Atypical hyperplasia		11.0	4.2–4.3
Atypical ductal hyperplasia	Has features similar to ductal carcinoma in situ but lacks the complete criteria for that diagnosis		
Atypical lobular hyperplasia	Defined by changes that are similar to lobular carcinoma in situ but lack the complete criteria for that diagnosis		
Nonproliferative	Normal, cysts, duct, ectasia, mild hyperplasia, fibroadenoma	1.2–2.6	0.9–1.0

g. Sclerosing adenosis increases the risk of breast cancer by approximately 70%, which justifies its inclusion among proliferative disease without atypia.

h. Fewer than 5% of women with a biopsy showing no proliferative changes develop breast cancer over the subsequent 25 years.

i. Nearly 40% of women with a family history of breast cancer and atypical hyperplasia subsequently develop breast cancer.

j. Estrogen replacement therapy lowers the risk of breast cancer in women with proliferative benign breast disease with or without atypia.

k. A history of proliferative benign breast disease is not a contraindication to estrogen replacement therapy.

II. **Family History of Breast Cancer**
   A. Genetic factors contribute to approximately 5% of all breast cancers and to 25% of cases diagnosed before age 30.
   B. Early-onset breast cancer is that which occurs before age 50.
   C. Additional information on the genetics of breast cancer is found in Chapter 3.

III. **Mammographic Parenchymal Pattern**
   A. In 1976, Wolfe proposed a subjective classification system for mammograms based solely on the radiographic appearance of the breast parenchyma.[16]
   B. Four parenchymal patterns (N1, P1, P2, DY) are associated with a stepwise increase in breast cancer risk.
      1. *Women showing the P1 pattern (mostly fat with less than 25% prominent duct pattern) or the DY pattern (sheetlike areas of increased density) are more likely to have a finding of lobular carcinoma in situ on breast biopsy.*
      2. *High densities with either the P2 (prominent linear and nodular ductal densities that occupy 25 to 100% of the breast area) or DY patterns are associated with odds ratios of 3.2 and 2.9, respectively, of developing breast cancer.*
      3. *Meta-analysis of multiple published studies shows a fivefold increase in risk for high-risk parenchymal patterns in prospective cohort studies and a twofold increase in retrospective case-control studies.*
      4. *High-risk patterns are more prevalent in countries with an increased incidence of breast cancer than in countries with a lower incidence of breast cancer.*
      5. *Breast densities in mammograms taken prior to a diagnosis of breast cancer and measured quantitatively using a computerized planimeter predict the subsequent risk of breast cancer.*[17]
         a. There is a linear increase in the risk of breast cancer with increasing breast density.
         b. The odds ratio was 4.3 for subsequent development of breast cancer for women in whom more than 65% of the breast area was dense.
         c. Women who had a quantitative breast density of 75% or greater by planimetry had a fivefold increased risk of breast cancer.
         d. In mammographic screening studies, 28% of the incident breast cancer cases are attributable to having 50% or greater breast density.
         e. This technique appears to be an independent measure of breast cancer risk although it has not gained wide acceptance in clinical practice.
      6. *Few correlations between the mammographic appearance and the associated histopathology have been published.*
      7. *In most women, mammographic parenchymal pattern is confounded by obesity, the normal aging process, and genetic factors.*

        8. *Mammographic lucency is closely associated with age, obesity, and large breast size.*[18]

        9. *The correlation of the mammographic pattern with the amount of breast parenchyma and the presence of fibrocystic changes is poor.*

   C. Because of these considerations, parenchymal pattern may not be an independent predictor of the risk of breast cancer.

IV.   **Environmental Factors**

   A. Few environmental exposures have been shown definitely to be associated with increased risk of breast cancer.

   B. Exposure to ionizing radiation is known to increase the risk.

      1. *Exposure to atomic bomb irradiation, chest fluoroscopy for tuberculosis, treatment of postpartum mastitis, diagnostic roentgenography for scoliosis, and therapeutic irradiation for either Hodgkin's disease or breast cancer are all associated with an increased risk of subsequent breast cancer.*

      2. *Relative risks vary from 1.2 to 2.4 and are related to both total dose and age at exposure, with younger women being at greater risk than older women.*

      3. *Individuals who are heterozygotes for the ataxia telangiectasia gene (ATM) make up about 1% of the general population.*

      4. *Female (ATM) heterozygotes who are exposed to ionizing radiation have nearly a sixfold increased risk of developing breast cancer compared with nonexposed controls.*

      5. *This observation raises concerns about the safety of mammographic screening in women who are (ATM) heterozygotes.*

      6. *There are no current public health recommendations regarding screening of these women.*

      7. *Recent cloning of the gene makes it possible that (ATM) heterozygotes can be identified, but a strategy to systematically identify and counsel these women remains to be defined.*

   C. There is no increased risk of breast cancer associated with exposire to electromagnetic fields (EMF).

References

1. Peto R, Boreham J, Clarke M, et al. UK and USA breast cancer deaths down 25% in year 2000 at ages 20–69 years. *Lancet* 2000;355:1822.

2. Gail MH, Brinton LA, Byar DP, et al. Projecting individualized probabilities of developing breast cancer for white females who are being examined annually. *J Natl Cancer Inst* 1989;81:1879–1886.

3. Kelsey JL, Berkowitz GS. Breast cancer epidemiology. *Cancer Res* 1988;48:5615–5623.

4. Kelsey JL, Gammon MD, John EM. Reproductive factors and breast cancer. *Epidemiol Rev* 1993;15:36–47.

5. Kelsey JL, Gammon MD. Epidemiology of breast cancer. *Epidemiol Rev* 1990;12:228–240.

6. Kelsey JL. A review of the epidemiology of human breast cancer. *Epidemiol Rev* 1979;1:74–109.

7. Vogel VG. Evaluation of risk and preventive approaches to breast cancer. In: Kavanagh J, Singletary SE, Einhorn N, DePetrillo AD, eds. *Cancer in Women.* Cambridge, MA: *Blackwell Scientific Publications, Inc;* 1998;58–91.

8. Dawson DA, Thompson GB. *Breast Cancer Risk Factors and Screening:* United States, 1987. National Center for Health Statistics. Vital Health Stat 10 (172), 1989.

9. Lippman ME, Swain SM. Endocrine-responsive cancers of humans. In: Wilson JD, Foster DW, eds. *Williams Textbook of Endocrinology.* 8th ed. Philadelphia, PA: WB Saunders Co; 1992:1577.

10. Hershcopf RJ, Bradlow HL. Obesity, diet, endogenous estrogens, and the risk of hormone-sensitive cancer. *Am J Clin Nutr* 1987;45:283–289.

11. Cauley JA, Gutai JP, Kuller LH, LeDonne D, Powell JG. The epidemiology of serum sex hormones in postmenopausal women. *Am J Epidemiol* 1989;129:1120–1131.

12. Ernster VL. The epidemiology of benign breast disease. *Epidemiol Rev* 1981;3:184–202.

13. Vogel VG. High risk populations as targets for breast cancer prevention trials. *Prev Med.* 1991;20:86–100.

14. London SJ, Connolly JL, Schnitt SJ, et al. A prospective study of benign breast disease and the risk of breast cancer. *JAMA* 1992;267:941–944.

15. Dupont WD, Parl FF, Hartman WH, et al. Breast cancer risk associated with proliferative disease and atypical hyperplasia. *Cancer* 1993;71:1258–1265.

16. Wolfe JN. Risk for breast cancer development determined by mammographic parenchymal pattern. *Cancer* 1976;37:2486–2492.

17. Saftlas AF, Hoover RN, Brinton LA, et al. Mammographic densities and risk of breast cancer. *Cancer* 1991;67:2833–2838.

18. Byrne C, Schairer C, Wolfe J, et al. Mammographic features and breast cancer risk: effects with time, age, and menopause status. *J Natl Cancer Inst* 1995;87:1622–1629.

chapter 2

Lifestyle Factors and Breast Cancer Risk

Deborah Davison, MSN, CRNP
NSABP Foundation, Inc.
Pittsburgh, PA

I.   While age-adjusted incidence of breast cancer has risen 1 to 2% per year over the past 50 years, mortality from breast cancer began to fall in North America in the mid-1990s. Multiple factors have been examined in epidemiological studies to explore these effects.

II. Diet
   A. Although there has been much speculation about the association between diet and breast cancer risk, to date, studies have not yielded firm evidence regarding the role of diet.
   B. Aspects of diet that have been studied most extensively include fat intake, vitamins, fruit and vegetable intake, and dietary fiber.
   C. Fat Intake
      1. *Case-control and prospective cohort studies have shown either weak or nonexistent associations between dietary fat and the risk of breast cancer.*
      2. *Analysis of seven prospective studies reveals no evidence of a positive association between total dietary fat intake and the risk of breast cancer.*[1]
      3. *Additionally, studies fail to show any association with regard to type of fat (saturated, monounsaturated, or polyunsaturated).*
      4. *There is also no association with fats derived from animal or vegetable sources.*
      5. *Age-adjusted incidence rates for breast cancer are highest in countries with the highest levels of dietary fat consumption.*
      6. *The Nurses' Health Study, a prospective evaluation of more than 90,000 registered nurses in the United States, found equal risks for breast cancer across all levels of dietary fat and fiber consumption for both premenopausal and postmenopausal women.*
         a. The explanation for these apparently conflicting observations may lie in the micronutrient components of the diets consumed rather than in the levels of total fat or calories.
         b. Some polyunsaturated fatty acids can serve as substrates for prostaglandin synthesis and are implicated in tumorigenesis.
            i.   Polyunsaturated fatty acids that have a double bond between the third and fourth carbon atoms (so-called omega-3 fatty acids) are competitive inhibitors of prostaglandin endoperoxidase synthetase.
            ii. Omega-3 fatty acids such as eicosapentanoic or docosahexanoic acids may act as dietary inhibitors of carcinogenesis.
            iii. This protective effect is suggested by the lower age-standardized breast cancer incidence rates from countries around the world where consumption of fish oil (a rich source of omega-3 fatty acids) is high.[2]
            iv. These data suggest a protective effect from fish oils, but additional studies in women are needed before dietary modification or supplementation can be recommended as a proven breast cancer prevention strategy.
      7. *Several studies, however, suggest that olive oil may provide some protective effect; further investigation is warranted.*

D. Increased soy protein consumption is significantly correlated with a reduction in the risk of breast cancer.
   1. *Asians eat diets rich in soybean products and have breast cancer death rates one-third to one-half those of women in the West.*
   2. *Foods made from soybeans contain large quantities of isoflavones, which are phytoestrogens with weak estrogen agonist activity and may interfere with the breast cancer-promoting effects of physiologic estrogen.*
   3. *It is not yet appropriate to suggest to women that they can significantly lower their risk of breast cancer by increasing their consumption of soybean products.*
E. Caffeine consumption does not increase the risk of breast cancer.

III. **Vitamins**
   A. Antioxidant vitamins may reduce the risk of cancer through their functions as free radical scavengers and as blockers of nitrosation reactions.[3]
   B. The epidemiological evidence demonstrating a significant relationship between either serum levels or dietary intake of Vitamins C and E and reduced risk of breast cancer is limited and inconsistent.[4]
   C. Review of published data provides no support for a protective effect from Vitamin E supplementation, even at high doses for long duration of use.[5-7]
   D. Prospective data do not indicate a protective effect from high doses of Vitamin C.
   E. Whether supplemental Vitamin A will reduce the risk of breast cancer for women with average dietary intakes of Vitamin A is not known.[5]
   F. Women should be cautioned not to exceed the recommended daily doses of vitamins that have known and potentially serious toxicities at higher doses.
   G. The Shanghai Breast Cancer Study, a case-control study, demonstrated a statistically significant reduction in breast cancer risk in women with the highest levels of folate intake.[8]
   H. This effect appears to be enhanced by the addition of the folate cofactors: Vitamin B6, Vitamin B12, and methionine.
   I. Some previous studies had indicated a benefit of folate in women who regularly consume alcohol.

IV. **Fruit and Vegetable Intake**
   A. A meta-analysis of 26 studies confirms an association between vegetable intake and breast cancer risk reduction.[9]
   B. This meta-analysis also indicates that there is a lesser association with fruit intake and risk reduction.
   C. Further prospective study is warranted in order to minimize other confounding dietary variables.

V.   **Dietary Fiber**
   A. Although high-fiber diets have been associated with reduced incidence of breast cancer in animals, studies in humans, including the Nurses' Health Study, have found no significant protective effect from dietary fiber.

VI. **Alcohol**
   A. There is increasing evidence that alcohol intake increases breast cancer risk. There are many mechanisms that could explain this relationship.[10–12] It may:
      1. *Induce increased levels of circulating estrogen.*
         a. There are major effects of alcohol on both estrogen production and metabolism.[13]
         b. It is not clear whether increased levels of bioavailable estradiol increase either the risk of breast cancer or the chance that a breast cancer will contain measurable estrogen receptors, but it is clear that alcohol may play some role.
      2. *Stimulate hepatic metabolism of carcinogens such as acetaldehyde.*
      3. *Facilitate transport of carcinogens into breast tissue.*
      4. *Stimulate pituitary production of prolactin.*
      5. *Modulate cell membrane integrity with an effect on carcinogenesis.*
      6. *Aid production of cytotoxic protein products.*
      7. *Impair immune surveillance.*
      8. *Interfere with DNA repair.*
      9. *Promote production of toxic congeners.*
      10. *Increase exposure to toxic oxidants.*
      11. *Reduce intake and bioavailability of protective nutrients.*
   B. Women who consume 2 to 5 drinks per day (30–60 grams) have a 41% higher risk of invasive breast cancer than cohorts that do not.[14]
      1. *This risk is similar for beer, wine, and liquor.*
      2. *The relative risk of one drink per day is 1.1, while the relative risk for three drinks per day is roughly 1.4.*
      3. *Meta-analysis of the published literature relating alcohol consumption and breast cancer shows strong evidence of a dose-response relationship with a very modest slope.*
      4. *The individual studies remain confounded by a number of biases.*
      5. *The data do not support a recommendation that women should abstain from alcohol to reduce their breast cancer risk.*
   C. Daily consumption of alcohol in first-degree relatives of women with breast cancer increases the risk of developing breast cancer (relative risk 2.45).[15]
   D. Women who are at increased risk for breast cancer and at low risk for heart disease may wish to consider limiting their alcohol consumption.

1. *The beneficial effects of light to moderate alcohol consumption on overall mortality must be taken into consideration before abstinence can be recommended as a breast cancer control strategy.*

2. *Women who are at increased risk for breast cancer and at low risk of heart disease may wish to consider limiting their alcohol consumption.*

VII. **Body Size**
   A. There is some evidence that body size (height, weight, and change in weight over time) may have a significant link to breast cancer risk.
   B. This may be related to estrogen exposure, but the relationship is likely to be much more complex.

VIII. **Height**
   A. Attained height is positively correlated with breast cancer rates, suggesting that childhood and adolescent energy intake may influence breast cancer rates decades later.
   B. Rapid growth rates accelerate the onset of menarche and result in greater attained height.
   C. The major predictors of age at menarche are weight, height, and body fat.
   D. Insulinlike growth factor-I (IGF-I) is directly involved in promotion of growth during childhood.
   E. Increased plasma levels of IGF-I in premenopausal women are associated with increased risk of breast cancer.

IX. **Weight and Weight Change**
   A. Although body weight is positively associated with the risk of developing breast cancer in postmenopausal women, a negative association between weight and breast cancer risk has been reported in premenopausal women.
   B. In Western populations, body weight is inversely related to the risk of premenopausal breast cancer.
   C. Obesity in premenopausal women is associated with decreased serum estradiol and progesterone, which is likely to be related to an increased frequency of anovulation.
   D. Recent studies demonstrate a significant link between weight gain and the risk of postmenopausal breast cancer.
      1. *Studies report either that a weight gain in adulthood is associated with increased risk of breast cancer or that the ratio of central to peripheral fat distribution affects risk.*
      2. *Weight gain after age 18 is significantly related to increased postmenopausal breast cancer risk (see Table 2.1).*
      3. *Whether this is related to endogenous estrogen production by adipose tissue remains speculative.*
      4. *The effect of obesity on other risk factors for breast cancer is not well studied with the exception of the association of obesity or large body size with early age at menarche.*

TABLE 2.1	Effect of Adult Weight on Breast Cancer Risk
Adult Weight Change after Age 18	**Relative Risk of Breast Cancer**
Loss of > 2 kg	1.1
± 2 kg	1.0
2.1–10 kg	1.2
10.1–20 kg	1.6
> 20 kg	2.0

Source: Huang Z, Hankinson SE, Colditz GA. Dual effects of weight and weight gain on breast cancer risk. *JAMA* 278:1407–1414, 1997.

E. Among women who never used hormone replacement therapy in the Nurses' Health Study, those who gained 25 kg or more after age 18 had double the risk of postmenopausal breast cancer compared to women who maintained their weight within 2 kg.[16]

F. It is not clear whether significant weight reduction has a substantial protective effect on breast cancer risk.

X. **Exercise**

A. Physical exercise may be biologically linked to breast cancer risk because strenuous physical activity is associated with an increase in luteal-phase defects, anovulation, and depressed serum estradiol levels in premenopausal women.[17]

B. It is not clear whether significant weight reduction has a substantial protective effect on breast cancer risk.

C. Studies of the role of exercise and physical activity in reducing breast cancer risk have yielded inconsistent results.[18]

D. Many of these studies are limited in their ability to control for other breast cancer risk factors.

E. There is difficulty in obtaining accurate measurement of physical activity and changes in level of activity over time.

F. Recent studies have attempted to evaluate the effect of lifetime physical activity.

G. Hypotheses to explain the role of exercise in breast cancer risk reduction include:

1. *Reduction in lifetime exposure to endogenous sex hormones.*
2. *Possible beneficial effect on body weight and fat distribution.*
3. *Reduction in levels of insulinlike growth factor-I.*
4. *Beneficial effect of moderate activity in enhancing the immune system.*

H. Physical activity appears to provide a protective effect in premenopausal women, which does not appear to be mediated by higher levels or longer duration of activity.[19]

I.   A recent case-control study by Friederich, et al. demonstrated a risk reduction in postmenopausal women who engaged in occupational and household activity.[20]

J.   This risk reduction was more prominent in women who were nondrinkers and nonsmokers.[21]

K.   Some recent studies have indicated that women who spend 1 to 3 hours per week in physical activity reduce their risk of breast cancer by 30% relative to inactive women.[22]

L.   It is not known if physical activity can reduce the risk associated with either genetic predisposition to breast cancer or proliferative benign breast disease.

M.   To date, the effect of exercise programs begun during the perimenopausal years is unstudied.

1.   *The hormonal consequences of physical activity and obesity are not well understood.*

2.   *Exercise may influence the prevalence of obesity, but large body mass has actually been associated with reductions in the risk of premenopausal breast cancer.*

3.   *Both the timing of weight change in adulthood and body fat distribution may be important determinants of risk.*

4.   *Moderate physical activity early in life can have a protective effect against the development of breast cancer.*

5.   *Various studies of different designs have shown nonsignificant protection afforded by physical activity or have shown unexpected increased risk among the most physically active women, either premenopausal or postmenopausal.*

6.   *Women with nonsedentary occupations may lower the risk of dying of breast cancer by approximately 15% but results have been inconsistent.*

7.   *Limitations of earlier studies:*
    a.   An inability to control for other breast cancer risk factors
    b.   Inaccurate measurement of physical activity
    c.   Failure to account for changes in activity over time

8.   *More recent studies with better methods do show that the average number of hours spent in physical exercise activities per week from menarche to early middle age is a significant predictor of reduced breast cancer risk.*
    a.   Women who spent 1 to 3 hours per week in physical activity reduced their risk of breast cancer by 30% relative to inactive women.
    b.   Those who exercised at least 4 hours per week reduced their risk by 50%.
    c.   The effect is greatest for women who have at least one child, and the effect is not lost among obese women.
    d.   The interaction of physical activity with other breast cancer risk factors is not yet clear.

9.   *We do not know if physical activity can reduce the risk associated with either genetic predisposition or proliferative benign breast disease.*

XI. **Environmental Exposures**
  A. There has been some concern that exposure to "environmental estrogens" (organochlorines) found in pesticides and industrial chemicals may contribute to increased risk of breast cancer.
  B. Studies, however, have failed to provide scientific evidence to support this concern.
      1. *A prospective study measured plasma levels of 1,1-dichloro-2,2-bis (p-chlorophenyl) ethylene (DDE) and polychlorinated biphenyls (PCBs) in breast cancer patients and matched controls. The median plasma levels of both DDE and PCBs were lower in the breast cancer patients than in the control group.*[23]
      2. *An analysis of five U.S. studies examining the role of organochlorines in breast cancer risk yielded no evidence of an association between plasma/serum levels of DDE and PCBs and increased risk of breast cancer.*[24]

XII. **Phytoestrogens**
  A. There are theories that intake of phytoestrogens (estrogenlike compounds derived from plants) may help to reduce the risk of breast cancer.
  B. Phytoestrogens are found in many food sources with the most prominent dietary source being soy.[25]
  C. Phytoestrogens may help to reduce the risk of breast cancer by:
      1. *Suppression or inhibition of normal estrogen production.*
      2. *Preventing tumor cells from dividing.*
      3. *Acting as an antioxidant.*
      4. *Preventing the formation of new blood vessels (antiangiogenesis).*
      5. *Increasing excretion of estrogen.*
  D. To date, there is no clear scientific evidence that increased intake of phytoestrogens will significantly reduce breast cancer risk.
  E. A case-control study demonstrated a statistically significant decrease in risk of breast cancer in subjects with a high intake of phytoestrogens.[26]
  F. These results, however, may be difficult to interpret fully as metabolism and excretion of phytoestrogens vary widely.
  G. Animal studies and some laboratory studies with estrogen receptor positive human breast cancer cells suggest that intake of low levels of phytoestrogens may actually stimulate growth of tumor cells, while high levels inhibit tumor growth.
  H. Unfortunately, there is currently not enough data to recommend the dose or frequency for phytoestrogen intake.
  I. Additionally, there is no information regarding the proper age at which exposure to phytoestrogens will confer the largest benefit (preadolescence versus lifetime exposure).
  J. Caution must be exercised when comparing Western and Asian populations with regard to theories about the benefit of

phytoestrogens as there are other factors (physical activity, weight patterns, diet) that vary significantly between these two groups.

XIII. Miscellaneous Factors

A. An increased number of lifetime ovulatory menstrual cycles increases the risk of breast cancer. This can occur with early age at menarche, late age at menopause, and/or few or no full-term pregnancies.

B. Lactation for two or more years decreases the lifetime risk of breast cancer by at least 50%, but this may be confined only to women with increased parity.

C. Spontaneous abortion does not increase the relative risk of breast cancer among parous women, while induced abortion may increase the risk of breast cancer in nulliparous women (RR = 1.3, 95% CI = 0.9–1.9).

D. The risk of breast cancer increases approximately 3% per year of delayed menopause (average age at menopause in North America is approximately 51 years).

References

1. Hunter DJ, Spiegelman D, Adami H, et al. Cohort studies of fat intake and the risk of breast cancer—a pooled analysis. *N Engl J Med* 1996;334:356–361.

2. Kaizer L, Boyd NF, Kriukov V, et al. Fish consumption and breast cancer risk: an ecological study. *Nutr Cancer* 1989;12:61–68.

3. Garland M, Willett WC, Manson JE, et al. Antioxidant micronutrients and breast cancer. *J Am Coll Nutr* 1993;12:400–411.

4. Hunter DJ, Manson JE, Colditz GA, et al. A prospective study of the intake of vitamins C, E, and A and the risk of breast cancer. *N Engl J Med* 1993;329:234–240.

5. Willett WC, Hunter DJ. Vitamin A and cancers of the breast, large bowel, and prostate: epidemiologic evidence. *Nutr Rev* 1994;52:S53–S59.

6. Willett WC. Diet and breast cancer. *J Intern Med* 2001;249:395–411.

7. Knekt P. Vitamin E and cancer: epidemiology. *Ann NY Acad Sci* 1992;669:269–279.

8. Shrubsole MJ, Jin F, Dai Q, et al. Dietary folate intake and breast cancer risk: results from the Shanghai Breast Cancer Study. *Cancer Res* 2001;61:7136–7141.

9. Gandini S, Merzenich H, Robertson C, Boyle P. Meta-analysis of studies on breast cancer risk and diet: the role of fruit and vegetable consumption and the intake of associated micronutrients. *Eur J Cancer* 2000;36:636–646.

10. Longnecker MP, Newcombe PA, Mittendorf R, et al. Risk of breast cancer in relation to lifetime alcohol consumption. *J Natl Cancer Inst* 1995;87:923–929.

11. Longnecker MP. Alcoholic beverage consumption in relation to risk of breast cancer: meta-analysis and review. *Cancer Causes Control* 1994;5:73–82.

12. Rosenberg L, Metzger LS, Palmer JR. Alcohol consumption and risk of breast cancer: a review of the epidemiologic evidence. *Am J Epidemiol* 1993;15:133–144.

13. Reichman ME, Judd JT, Longscope C, et al. Effects of alcohol consumption on plasma and urinary hormone concentrations in premenopausal women. *J Natl Cancer Inst* 1993;85:722–727.

14. Smith-Warner SA, Spiegelman D, Yaun S, et al. Alcohol and breast cancer in women: a Pooled analysis of cohort studies. *JAMA* 1998;279:535–540.

15. Vachon CM, Cerhan JR, Vierkant RA, Sellers TA. Investigation of an interaction of alcohol intake and family history on breast cancer risk in the Minnesota Breast *Cancer* Family Study. *Cancer* 2001;92:240–248.

16. Huang Z, Hankinson SE, Colditz GA. Dual effects of weight and weight gain on breast cancer risk. *JAMA* 278:1407–1414, 1997.

17. Frisch RE, Wyshak G, Albright NL, et al. Lower prevalence of breast cancer and cancers of the reproductive system among former college athletes compared to non-athletes. *Br J Cancer* 1985;52:885–891.

18. Albanes D, Blair A, Taylor PR. Physical activity and risk of cancer in the NHANES I population. *Am J Public Health* 1989;79:744–750.

19. Verloop J, Rookus MA, van der Kooy K, van Leeuwen FE. Physical activity and breast cancer risk in women aged 20–54 years. *J Natl Cancer Inst* 2000;92:128–135.

20. Friederich CM, Bryant HE, Courneya KS. Case-control study of lifetime physical activity and breast cancer risk. *Am J Epidemiol* 2001;154:336–347.

21. Vena JE, Graham S, Zielezny M, et al. Occupational exercise and risk of cancer. *Am J Clin Nutr* 1987;45:318–327.

22. Bernstein L, Henderson BE, Hanisch R, et al. Physical exercise and reduced risk of breast cancer in young women. *J Natl Cancer Inst* 1994;86:1403–1408.

23. Hunter DJ, Hankinson SE, Laden F, et al. Plasma organochlorine levels and the risk of breast cancer. *N Engl J Med* 1997;337:1253–1258.

24. Laden F, Collman G, Iwamoto K, et al. 1,1-dichloro-2,2-bis(p-chloro-phenyl)ethylene and poly-chorinated biphenyls and breast cancer: combined analysis of five U.S. studies. *J Natl Cancer Inst* 2001;93:768–776.

25. Barnes S, Peterson G, Grubbs C, et al. Potential role of dietary isoflavones in the prevention of cancer. In: Jacobs MM, ed. *Diet and Cancer: Markers, Prevention, and Treatment*. New York: Plenum; 1994:135.

26. Ingram D, Sanders K, Kolybaba M, Lopez D. Case-control study of phytoestrogens and breast cancer. *Lancet* 1997;350:990–994.

chapter 3

Genetics of Breast Cancer

Darcy L. Thull, MS
Dana Farengo-Clark, MS, MS
Magee-Womens Hospital/University of Pittsburgh
Cancer Institute
Cancer Genetics Program
Magee-Womens Hospital
Pittsburgh, PA

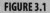 **FIGURE 3.1** Heterogeneity of Breast Cancer

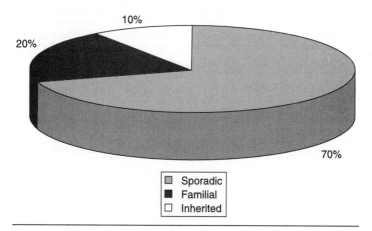

10%

20%

70%

- Sporadic
- Familial
- Inherited

I. **Breast Cancer Etiology**
   A. All cancer is due to changes (mutations) in the DNA.
   B. Seventy to 80% of breast cancer is sporadic or occurs by chance as a result of multiple acquired (somatic) genetic mutations in a given breast cell.
   C. About 15 to 20% of breast cancer is familial.
      1. *Breast cancer occurs within the context of a positive family history of the disease in several family members.*
      2. *These cases are likely the result of multiple genetic and shared environmental factors working together over time.*
      3. *Because of the genetic component, there is an increased risk for breast cancer in other family members which can be quantified by the epidemiologic risk models[1, 2] that are discussed in Chapter 11.*
   D. Five to 10% of breast cancer occurs as the result of a hereditary predisposition caused by a mutation in a single cancer susceptibility gene, which confers considerable risk (Figure 3.1).

II. **Features of a Hereditary Susceptibility to Breast Cancer (a more detailed description is provided in Chapter 11).**
   A. Breast cancer in two or more relatives from the same lineage
   B. Early age at diagnosis (< 50 years of age)
   C. Bilateral disease
   D. Multiple primary tumors (breast and ovarian)
   E. Group of features consistent with a genetic syndrome
   F. Male breast cancer
   G. Ashkenazi Jewish ancestry
   H. A relative with a mutation in a known cancer susceptibility gene

TABLE 3.1	Hereditary Syndromes, Associated Genes and Proportion of Hereditary Breast Cancer Cases

Syndrome	Associated Genes	Proportion of Hereditary Breast Cancer Cases (%)
Site-specific breast cancer (Families with ≥4 cases of breast cancer)	BRCA1 BRCA2	50[1] 30[1]
Hereditary Breast-Ovarian Cancer (HBOC)	BRCA1 BRCA2	70[1] 20[1]
Cowden syndrome (CS)	PTEN	<1
Li-Fraumeni syndrome (LFS)	TP53	<1[2]
Ataxia-Telangiectasia heterozygotes (A-T)	ATM	unknown
Peutz-Jeghers syndrome (PJS)	STK11	<1
Other	unknown	~20

1. Ford D, et al. Genetic heterogeneity and penetrance analysis of the BRCA1 and BRCA2 genes in breast cancer families. The Breast Cancer Linkage Consortium. Am J Hum Genet 1998;62:676–689.

2. Easton DF, et al. Genetic linkage analysis in familial breast and ovarian cancer: results from 214 families. The Breast Cancer Linkage Consortium. Am J Hum Genet 1993;52:678–701.

III. **Hereditary Syndromes Predisposing to Breast Cancer (Table 3.1)**

IV. **BRCA1 and BRCA2 Genes**
   A. Clinical Summary
      1. *Hereditary Breast and Ovarian Cancer syndrome (HBOC)*
         a. HBOC is characterized by several generations of women affected with breast and/or ovarian cancer.
         b. Hallmark features include early-onset breast cancer (<50 years), increased incidence of bilateral disease, breast and ovarian cancer in the same individual, and occasionally male breast cancer and other cancers.
      2. *Site-specific breast cancer*
         a. Criteria for a site-specific breast cancer family include four or more cases of female breast cancer diagnosed at less than 60 years of age without any cases of ovarian cancer.[3] Male breast cancer might or might not be included within these families.
   B. Inheritance, Prevalence, Location, and Function
      1. *Breast Cancer 1 Gene (BRCA1)*
         a. Autosomal Dominant (AD) transmission
            i.   The predisposition occurs in successive generations of the same lineage, but not all carriers of the genetic mutation will develop cancer (reduced penetrance).
            ii. Both males and females can inherit the cancer predisposition.
            iii. When a parent carries the predisposition, each child has a 50% chance to inherit the cancer susceptibility.
         b. The mutation frequency likely lies somewhere between 1 in 833[4] and 1 in 152.[5]

   c. Location and structure
- i. Large gene comprising 100 kb of genomic DNA on chromosome 17q21, consisting of 24 exons.[6]
- ii. Cancer risks vary with position of the mutation within the gene.
  - Truncating mutations in the C-terminal end of the coding regions are associated with an increased risk for early-onset breast cancer.[7]
  - Mutations in the 5' end of the gene are associated with a higher risk of ovarian cancer than mutations in the 3' end of the gene.[8]
- iii. The protein has a zinc-binding RING finger domain at the N-terminus and a BRCT domain at the C-terminus, both normally involved in protein-protein interactions.
- iv. The RING finger specifically binds with the protein BARD1 (BRCA1 Associated Ring Domain).[9]

   d. Function
- i. Initially identified as a tumor suppressor gene, as wild-type, allele is deleted in tumors of BRCA1 mutation carriers (Loss of Heterozygosity or LOH).
- ii. May play a role in cell cycle regulation and DNA repair.
  - BRCT domain binds TP53 and other proteins that are involved in cell cycle regulation or gene expression.[10]
  - BRCA1 interacts with the RAD51 protein, which has a role in DNA repair and recombination.[11]

2. *Breast Cancer 2 Gene (BRCA2)*

   a. Autosomal Dominant transmission with reduced penetrance.

   b. The mutation frequency of BRCA2 has been reported as 1 in 1136.[3]

   c. Location
- i. Large gene comprising 70 kb of genomic DNA on chromosome 13q12 consisting of 27 exons without known protein motifs.[12]
- ii. Truncating mutations in families with a high proportion of ovarian cancer are clustered in a 3.3 kb portion of exon 11, named the ovarian cancer cluster region (OCCR).[13]

   d. Function
- i. Identified as a tumor suppressor gene, as both alleles must be nonfunctioning for tumor formation.
- ii. Also interacts with the RAD51 protein and is involved in DNA damage repair pathways.[14]

C. Average Age of Breast Cancer Diagnosis

1. *Breast cancer in known mutation carriers typically occurs at an earlier age (<45 years), as compared to people with sporadic breast cancer.*

2. *Penetrance of BRCA1/2 mutations by age was reported by Ford and colleagues[3] (Table 3.2).*

3. *Breast cancer age at diagnosis was older for BRCA2 mutation carriers than for BRCA1 carriers (50% of BRCA1 carriers diagnosed before 40 years; 30% of BRCA2 carriers diagnosed before 40 years).[3]*

D. Lifetime Risks for Cancer in BRCA1 and BRCA2 Mutations Carriers (Table 3.3)

1. *The cancer risks may be overestimated due to highly selected families with multiple cases of breast and/or ovarian cancer from which the data were generated.*

| TABLE 3.2 | Penetrance of BRCA1 and BRCA2 Mutations[1] | | | |

Age	BRCA1		BRCA2	
	HBOC families (%)	Breast only families (%)	HBOC families (%)	Breast only families (%)
30	3.6	3.6	4.6	4.6
40	18	18	12	12
50	57	49	46	45
60	75	64	61	59
70	83	71	86	83

1. Ford D, et al. Genetic heterogeneity and penetrance analysis of the BRCA1 and BRCA2 genes in breast cancer families. The Breast Cancer Linkage Consortium. Am J Hum Genet. 1998;62:676–689.

TABLE 3.3	Lifetime Risks (%) for Cancer to age 70 in BRCA1 and BRCA2 Mutation Carriers	
Site	BRCA1(%)	BRCA2(%)
Breast	50–85[1]	50–85[1]
Contralateral Breast	64[2]	50[3]
Ovary	20–40[1]	10–27[2]
Male Breast	Low	6[4]
Pancreatic		2–3[3]
Prostate		8[3]
Other	Colon[1*]	Stomach, melanoma, gallbladder/bile duct[3]

*Increased risk has not been identified in subsequent studies.

1. Ford D, et al. Risks of cancer in BRCA1-mutation carriers. Breast Cancer Linkage Consortium. Lancet. 1994;343:692–695.

2. Ford D, et al. Genetic heterogeneity and penetrance analysis of the BRCA1 and BRCA2 genes in breast cancer families. The Breast Cancer Linkage Consortium. Am J Hum Genet. 1998;62:676–689.

3. Cancer risks in BRCA2 mutation carriers. The Breast Cancer Linkage Consortium. J Natl Cancer Inst. 1999;91:1310–1316.

4. Easton DF, et al. Cancer risks in two large breast cancer families linked to BRCA2 on chromosome 13q12-13. Am J Hum Genet. 1997;61:120–128.

2. Penetrance is likely dependent upon the specific mutation and the interactions of the BRCA1 and BRCA2 genes with other genetic and environmental factors yet to be determined.

E. BRCA Founder Mutations

1. Specific gene mutations that can be traced back to a common ancestor and are more prevalent in a given population as a result of migration patterns or geographic or social isolation.

TABLE 3.4	**Cancer Risks Associated with the BRCA1 and BRCA2 Ashkenazi Jewish Founder Mutations[1]**
Site	***BRCA1*** **(185delAG and 5382insC) and *BRCA2* (6174insT)**
Breast	56% (95% CI, 40–73%)
Ovary	16% (95% CI, 6–28%)
Prostate	16% (95% CI, 4–30%)

1. Struewing JP, et al. *The risk of cancer associated with specific mutations of BRCA1 and BRCA2 among Ashkenazi Jews.* N Engl J Med 1997;336:1401–1408.

     2. *Founder mutations have been identified in several populations (Icelandic, French Canadian, Finnish, and Dutch), but none has been studied as extensively as the Ashkenazi (Central and Eastern European) Jewish population.*

     3. *Three founder mutations, two in BRCA1 (185delAG and 5382insC) and one in BRCA2 (6174delT), are prevalent in the Ashkenazi population.*

        a. The combined prevalence of these recurrent mutations is 1 in 40 (2.5%).[15]

        b. Cancer risks associated with the three founder mutations (Table 3.4).

  F. Histopathology of BRCA1- and BRCA2-Associated Breast Cancer

     1. *Breast cancers associated with BRCA1 and BRCA2 mutations differ from each other and from sporadic breast cancers in their histopathologic features.*

     2. *When compared to sporadic breast cancers, BRCA1-associated tumors show the following features:*

        a. Higher proportion of medullary or atypical medullary carcinomas[16]

        b. Higher tumor grade[16]

        c. Increased tubule formation[17]

        d. Higher mitotic count[17]

        e. Higher frequency of ER/PR negativity[18]

        f. Lower expression of Her2-neu[19]

     3. *When compared to sporadic breast cancers, BRCA2-associated tumors show the following features:*

        a. Higher tumor grade[16]

        b. Decreased tubule formation[17]

        c. Decreased mitotic count[17]

        d. Higher frequency of ER/PR positivity

  G. Survival of Breast Cancer Patients with BRCA1 and BRCA2 Mutations

     1. *Survival of BRCA1-associated breast cancer (cases) compared to sporadic breast cancer (controls)*

        a. Survival is better than had been predicted based on histopathologic features.

        b. Older studies (1994–1996), done by linkage analysis, showed cases to have better prognosis than controls.[21,22]

TABLE 3.5	Frequency of BRCA1 Mutations in Young Breast Cancer Patients			
Study	Age at diagnosis	Family history	Number of cases (women with breast cancer)	Mutations identified
Fitzgerald et al., 1996[1]	Before 30 years	33% had FDR	30	4 (13%)
	Before 40 years (Ashkenazi Jewish)	51% had FDR/SDR	39	8 (21%) Only 185 delAG examined
Malone et al., 1998[2]	Before 35 years	Unselected for family history	193	12 (6.2%)
	Before 45 years	Unselected for family history	208	15 (7.2%)
Couch et al., 1997[3]	Before 40 years	Unselected for family history	94	12 (13%)

FDR = First-degree relative affected with breast cancer

SDR = Second-degree relative affected with breast cancer

1. Fitzgerald MG, et al. Germ-line BRCA1 mutations in Jewish and non-Jewish women with early-onset breast cancer. [see comments]. N Engl J Med. 1996;334:143–149.

2. Malone KE, et al. BRCA1 mutations and breast cancer in the general population: analyses in women before age 35 years and in women before age 45 years with first-degree family history. JAMA. 1998;279:922–929.

3. Couch FJ, et al. BRCA1 mutations in women attending clinics that evaluate the risk of breast cancer. [see comments]. N Engl J Med. 1997;336:1409–1415.

    c. More recent studies, based on mutation status, have shown no significant differences in overall survival.[23,24]

    d. Some studies suggest significantly inferior overall survival in cases.[25,26]

2. *Survival of BRCA2-associated breast cancer (cases) compared to sporadic breast cancer (controls)*

    a. Very few studies are available for BRCA2 carriers; small numbers of cases.

    b. Most studies show no difference in overall survival between cases and controls.[27–29]

    c. Several studies show cases have significantly worse survival.[30,31]

H. Mutation Frequency in Young Women

1. *Women affected with breast cancer at an early age (<50 years) are thought to have an increased risk to carry a genetic alteration in BRCA1/2.*

2. *Studies focusing on carrier frequency in young women have a wide range of estimates; however, carrier frequency is thought to be small (Tables 3.5 and 3.6).*

TABLE 3.6	Frequency of BRCA1 and BRCA2 Mutations in Young Breast Cancer Patients			
Study	Age at diagnosis	Family history	Number of cases (women with breast cancer)	Mutations identified
Malone et al., 2000[1]	Before 35 years	Unselected for family history	203	12 (5.9%) in BRCA1 7 (3.4%) in BRCA2
	Before 45 years	FDR diagnosed before 45 years	225	16 (7.1%) in BRCA1 11 (4.9%) in BRCA2
Peto et al., 1999[2]	Before 36 years	6.7% had FDR	254	9 (3.5%) in BRCA1 6 (2.4%) in BRCA2
	36–45 years	9% had FDR	363	7 (1.9%)in BRCA1 8 (9.1%) in BRCA2

FDR = First-degree relative affected with breast cancer
SDR = Second-degree relative affected with breast cancer

1. Malone KE, et al. Frequency of BRCA1/BRCA2 mutations in a population-based sample of young breast carcinoma cases. Cancer. 2000;88:1393–1402.

2. Peto J, et al. Prevalence of BRCA1 and BRCA2 gene mutations in patients with early-onset breast cancer. J Natl Cancer Inst. 1999;91:943–949.

I. Genetic Testing

1. Genetic testing is clinically available for BRCA1 and BRCA2 by full DNA sequencing.

2. Ideally testing should start with an individual affected with breast or ovarian cancer to determine if a mutation can be identified.

3. Full sequencing can identify approximately 63% of mutations in BRCA1 and BRCA2.[3]

4. Testing in individuals of certain ethnic backgrounds (Ashkenazi Jewish, Dutch, and Icelandic) is more targeted and can detect almost 100% of founder mutations.

J. Management of BRCA Mutations Carriers (Figure 3.2)

V. Cowden Syndrome (CS) or Multiple Hamartoma Syndrome
  A. Inheritance, Prevalence, Location, and Function

1. Autosomal Dominant with variable expression (not all affected individuals manifest all or the same features); most affected individuals (>90%) manifest features by their twenties.[32–34]

FIGURE 3.2   Management of BRCA1/2 Mutations Carriers

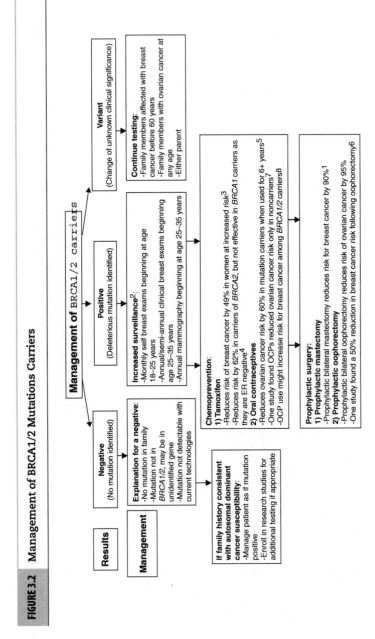

Management of BRCA1/2 carriers

Results

Negative
(No mutation identified)

Positive
(Deleterious mutation identified)

Variant
(Change of unknown clinical significance)

Management

Explanation for a negative:
-No mutation in family
-Mutation not in
BRCA1/2, may be in
unidentified gene
-Mutation not detectable with
current technologies

**If family history consistent
with autosomal dominant
cancer susceptibility:**
-Manage patient as if mutation
positive
-Enroll in research studies for
additional testing if appropriate

Increased surveillance[2]:
-Monthly self breast exams beginning at age
18–25 years
-Annual/semi-annual clinical breast exams beginning
age 25–35 years
-Annual mammography beginning at age 25–35 years

Chemoprevention:
1) Tamoxifen
-Reduces risk of breast cancer by 49% in women at increased risk[3]
-Reduces risk by 62% in carriers of BRCA2, but not effective in BRCA1 carriers as
they are ER negative[4]
2) Oral contraceptives
-Reduces ovarian cancer risk by 60% in mutation carriers when used for 6+ years[5]
-One study found OCPs reduced ovarian cancer risk only in noncarriers[7]
-OCP use might increase risk for breast cancer among BRCA1/2 carriers[8]

Prophylactic surgery:
1) Prophylactic mastectomy
-Prophylactic bilateral mastectomy reduces risk for breast cancer by 90%[1]
2) Prophylactic oophorectomy
-Prophylactic bilateral oophorectomy reduces risk of ovarian cancer by 95%
-One study found a 50% reduction in breast cancer risk following oophorectomy[6]

Continue testing:
-Family members affected with breast
cancer before 60 years
-Family members with ovarian cancer at
any age
-Either parent

1. Hartmann LC, et al. Efficacy of bilateral prophylactic mastectomy in women with a family history of breast cancer. N.Engl.J Med 1999;340:77–84.

2. Burke W, et al. Recommendations for follow-up care of individuals with an inherited predisposition to cancer. JAMA 1997;277:997–1003.

3. Fisher B, et al. Tamoxifen for prevention of breast cancer: report of the National Surgical Adjuvant Breast and Bowel Project P-1 Study. J Natl Cancer Inst 1998;90:1371–1388.

4. King MC, et al. Tamoxifen and breast cancer incidence among women with inherited mutations in BRCA1 and BRCA2. JAMA 2001;286:2251–2256.

5. Narod S, Risch H, Moslehi R, et al. Oral contraceptives and the risk of hereditary ovarian cancer. N Engl J Med 1998;339:424–428.

6. Rebbeck TR, et al. Breast cancer risk after bilateral prophylactic oophorectomy in BRCA1 mutation carriers. J Natl Cancer Inst. 1999;91:1475–1479.

7. Modan B, et al. Parity, oral contraceptives, and the risk of ovarian cancer among carriers and noncarriers of a BRCA1 or BRCA2 mutation. N Engl J Med. 2001;345:235–240.

8. Ursin G, et al. Does oral contraceptive use increase the risk of breast cancer in women with BRCA1/BRCA2 mutations more than in other women? Cancer Research 1997;57:3678–3681.

TABLE 3.7	Common Manifestations of Cowden Syndrome

Mucocutaneous lesions (90–100%)
- Trichilemmomas (hamartomas of the hair follicles)
- Acral keratoses
- Verucoid or papillomatous papules

Thyroid Abnormalities (50–67%)
- Goiter
- Adenoma
- Cancer 3–10%

Breast lesions
- Fibroadenomas/fibrocystic breast disease (76% of affected females)
- Adenocarcinoma (25–50% of affected females)

Gastrointestinal lesions (40%)
- Hamartomatous polyps

Macrocephaly (38%)

Genito-urinary Abnormalities (44% females)
- Uterine leiomyoma (multiple, early onset)

Eng C. Cowden Syndrome. *Journal of Genetic Counseling* 1997;6:181–191.

    2. CS is estimated to occur in 1 in 200,000 people, but this may be an underestimate due to incomplete ascertainment.[32]

    3. The gene was mapped to 10q22-23 and subsequently identified as PTEN.[32]

    4. PTEN acts as a tumor suppressor gene through cell cycle arrest or apoptosis or both.[33,34]

  B. Clinical Features of CS

    1. Cowden syndrome is associated with multiple hamartoma and an increased risk for benign and malignant breast and thyroid tumors.

    2. Common Manifestations (Table 3.7)

  C. Diagnostic Criteria (Table 3.8)

  D. Associated Cancer Risks (Table 3.9)

VI. Li-Fraumeni Syndrome (LFS)

  A. Inheritance, Prevalence, Gene Location, and Gene Function

    1. Autosomal Dominant, highly penetrant.

    2. LFS is very rare.

    3. Germline mutations in the TP53, tumor suppressor gene located on chromosome 17p13 were recognized to cause LFS by Malkin and colleagues;[35] however, genetic heterogeneity (other genes may cause LFS) may be a feature of LFS.[36]

    4. TP53 plays a critical role in cell cycle control via recognition of DNA damage and programmed cell death (apoptosis).[37]

  B. Clinical Summary

    1. LFS is characterized by earlyonset breast cancer, soft tissue sarcomas, leukemia, brain tumors, and adrenocortical carcinomas.[38]

TABLE 3.8	International Cowden Consortium Operational Criteria for the Diagnosis of Cowden Syndrome (Version 2000)

Pathognomonic Criteria
  Mucocutaneous lesions
    Facial Trichilemmoma
    Acral Keratoses
    Papillomatous papules
    Mucosal lesions
Major Criteria
  Breast Cancer
  Thyroid Cancer (nonmedullary), especially follicular carcinoma
  Macrocephaly ($\geq$95%)
  Lhermitte-Duclos disease or LDD (cerebellar dysplastic gangliocytoma)
  Endometrial carcinoma
Minor Criteria
  Other thyroid lesions (e.g., adenoma or multinodular goiter)
  Mental retardation (IQ$\leq$75)
  GI hamartomas
  Fibrocystic breast disease
  Lipomas
  Fibromas
  GU tumors (e.g., renal cell carcinoma, uterine fibroids) or malformation
Operational Diagnosis in a Person
1. Mucocutaneous lesions alone if there are:
  a. six or more facial papules, of which three or more must be trichilemmoma, or
  b. cutaneous facial papules and oral mucosal papillomatosis, or
  c. oral mucosal papillomatosis and acral keratoses, or
  d. palmoplantar keratoses, six or more
2. Two major criteria, but one must be macrocephaly or Lhermitte-Duclos disease
3. One major and three minor criteria
4. Four minor criteria
Operational diagnosis in a Family Where One Individual is Diagnosed With Cowden Syndrome
1. The pathognomonic criterion(ia)
2. Any one major criterion with or without minor criteria
3. Two minor criteria

    2. *Other hallmark features include unusually early age at cancer diagnosis (childhood and early adulthood) and multiple primary tumors in one individual.*

  C. Diagnostic Definition of LFS
    1. *Index case with sarcoma <45 years and*
      a. a first-degree (parents, siblings, children) relative having sarcoma, breast cancer, primary brain tumor, adrenocortical carcinoma, or leukemia diagnosed <45 years, and
      b. cancer diagnosed in a first- or second-degree (grandparents, aunts, uncles, niece, nephew) relative <45 years or a sarcoma at any age.[39]
    2. *A less strict definition for "Li-Fraumeni-like" families has been proposed by Birch and colleagues for families that share some but not all of the features associated with LFS.*[40]

  D. LFS Cancer Risks
    1. *LFS likely accounts for <1% of all breast cancer cases*[41], *however, within LFS kindred, breast cancer accounts for up to 30% of all tumors and occurs at an average age of 36 years.*[42,43]

TABLE 3.9	Cowden Syndrome Associated Cancer Risks
Site	**Malignant Tumors**
Female breast*	25–50%[1,2]
Thyroid	10%[3]
Lhermitte-Duclos disease	Not clearly known
Endometrial	Not clearly known, possibly 5–10%[4]
Other occasionally seen tumors	Skin cancers, renal cell carcinoma, and brain tumors

*Male breast cancer has been reported in PTEN-positive men.[5]

1. Brownstein M, Wolk M, Bikowski JB. Cowden's disease: a cutaneous marker of breast cancer. Cancer 1978;41:2393–2398.

2. Starink T, van der Veen JP, Arwert F, et al. The Cowden syndrome: a clinical and genetic study in 21 patients. Clin Genet 1986;29:222–233.

3. Eng C. Cowden syndrome. J Genet Counsel 1997;6:181–191.

4. Eng C. Will the real Cowden syndrome please stand up: revised diagnostic criteria. J Med Genet 2000;37:828–830.

5. Fackenthal J, Marsh DJ, Richardson AL, et al. Male breast cancer in Cowden syndrome patients with germline PTEN mutations. J Med Genet 2001;38:159–164.

2. Overall, the cancer risk for mutation carriers is estimated to be 50% by age 30 years and 90% by age 70 years.

3. Breast cancer risk has been estimated to be about 50% by age 50 years in female mutation carriers.

4. In a study of 24 LFS families, the average risk for a second malignancy was 57% at 30 years following the first diagnosis.[44]

E. Genetic testing is available on a limited clinical basis and consists of direct gene testing that detects mutations in approximately 70% of affected families diagnosed by the strict clinical definition and 22% of the Li-Fraumeni-like families.[45]

F. Management

1. Agreement on specific surveillance strategies is lacking due to the spectrum of tumors associated with LFS and the concern that radiation exposure may increase the risk for tumor development.

2. A complete annual physical exam is warranted and persistent health complaints should be investigated thoroughly.

3. Varley and colleagues advocate annual breast cancer screening in women with LFS starting at age 20 years to include a breast examination by a specialist with or without ultrasound evaluation.[46]

4. The use of breast MRI may become part of the screening program for women with LFS as more data regarding the efficacy of this technology for the diagnosis of breast cancer are collected.

VII. **Ataxia-Telangiectasia (A-T)**
   A. Inheritance, Prevalence, Gene Location, and Gene Function
      1. *Autosomal recessive.*
         a. Two copies of the mutated gene are necessary for an individual to be affected, and
         b. Carrier (individual having one normal gene and one mutated gene) parents have a 25% chance, with each pregnancy to have an affected child.
      2. *A-T occurs in about 1 out of 40,000 to 1 out of 100,000 live births.*[47]
      3. *Heterozygote (carrier) frequency is estimated at 1 in 100.*[48]
      4. *The A-T gene, ATM (ataxia telangiectasia mutated), is located on chromosome 11q23.*[49]
      5. *ATM is thought to participate in the processing of DNA damage, maintaining genome stability and cell cycle regulation.*[50]
   B. Clinical Summary
      1. *ATM homozygosity results in cerebellar ataxia, immune defects, telangiectases, radiosensitivity, and predisposition to malignancy (especially lymphoma and leukemia).*[51]
      2. *Obligate ATM heterozygotes may have increased radiosensitivity*[52] *and breast cancer predisposition.*[48]
      3. *ATM heterozygosity may account for about 8% of all breast cancer cases.*[48]
   C. Breast Cancer Risks
      1. *Obligate ATM heterozygotes.*
         a. Based on a study of 110 families with A-T, Swift and colleagues estimated a relative risk of 6.8 for breast cancer in female heterozygotes as compared to female family members related by marriage.[48]
         b. A prospective study of 161 families with A-T determined a relative risk of 5 for breast cancer in women carriers of ATM as compared to noncarriers.[53]
         c. A number of additional studies suggest a threefold to fourfold increased risk of breast cancer in female relatives of A-T patients, especially those known to be heterozygous carriers (mothers of A-T patients) as compared to noncarriers.[54–56]
      2. *ATM studies in young breast cancer patients, not selected for a family history of A-T, have failed to identify obvious gene mutations, suggesting that ATM does not play a large role in early-onset breast cancer.*[47,51]
   D. Genetic testing for ATM mutations is available on a limited clinical basis, but is not generally used to identify heterozygotes due to the cost, inefficiency of current testing methods, and the uncertain usefulness of a positive result.
   E. No specific management recommendations are suggested for ATM heterozygotes; however due to the concern for increased radiosensitivity in ATM carriers, the risks and benefits of heightened mammography need to be weighed.

VIII. **Peutz-Jeghers Syndrome (PJS)**
   A. Inheritance, Incidence, Gene Location, and Gene Function
      1. *Autosomal dominant.*

    2. PJS is a hamartoma syndrome that is estimated to occur in 1 in 8,300 to 29,000 live births;[57] however, about 40% of the cases are due to new mutations and represent the first case of PJS in the family.[58]

    3. PJS is caused by mutations in the STK11 (LKB1) gene, which encodes a serine threonine kinase and is located on chromosome 19p13.3.[59,60]

    4. Loss of heterozygosity (LOH) for markers near the STK11 gene in 70% of tumors from PJS patients provides evidence that STK11 is a tumor suppressor gene.[61]

B. Clinical Summary

    1. Hallmark features of PJS are diffuse harmatomatous polyps of the GI tract (especially small bowel) and melanin spots on the lips, buccal mucosa, and skin that all fade in adulthood with the exception of the pigmentation of the buccal mucosa.[58]

    2. PJS is associated with increased relative risk for both gastrointestinal and extraintestinal malignancies.[62,63]

    3. Boardman and colleagues found a mean age of 39.4 years at the time of cancer diagnosis.[62]

C. Cancer risks have been estimated to be 9 to 18 times higher than in the general population in PJS patients[62,63] with the most frequently reported malignancies occurring in the colon (mean age 45 years) and breast (mean age 44 years).[58]

D. Associated Malignancies[62,63]

    1. GI (stomach, colon, pancreas, small bowel)

    2. Breast

    3. Thyroid

    4. Lung

    5. Uterine

E. Other neoplasms have been reported and include:[58]

    1. Ovarian sex-cord tumors with annular tubules

    2. Sertoli cell tumors

F. Genetic Testing

    1. Clinical genetic testing for mutations in the STK11 (LKB1) gene is available on a limited clinical basis.

    2. Various methodologies have detected mutations in 50 to 60% of PJS patients.[64,65]

G. Management of PJS primarily focuses on treatment of symptomatic polyps; however, because of the increased cancer risk, especially GI, breast, and gynecologic, Vasen has proposed the surveillance measures described in Table 3.10.[58]

IX. **Guidelines for Cancer Susceptibility Testing as Published by the American Society for Clinical Oncology**[66]

A. Components of Genetic Testing

    1. Pretest and posttest counseling

    2. Informed consent

    3. Consider testing within the context of outcome studies

TABLE 3.10	Suggested cancer surveillance for PJS[1]	
Screening	**Time Interval**	**Age**
Gastroduodenoscopy and small bowel follow-through	Every 2–5 years	From age 15 to 20 years
Colonoscopy	Every 2–5 years	>20 years
Mammography and gynecologic examination	Regular	Starting 30–35 years

1. Vasen H, Clinical diagnosis and management of hereditary colorectal cancer syndromes. J Clin Oncol 2000. 18(21s): 81S–92S.

B. Indications for Testing
   1. A family history that is suspicious for a hereditary cancer predisposition or a history of early onset disease.
      a. For BRCA1 and BRCA2 testing, an a priori mutation risk of >10% is indicated.
      b. See Chapter 11.
   2. Adequate results interpretation is possible (in general, this implies initiating testing in an affected individual).
   3. The results will affect medical management.
C. Disease Categories for Predisposition Testing
   1. **Group 1–** "Tests for families with well-defined hereditary syndromes for which either a positive or negative result will change medical care, and for which genetic testing may be considered part of the standard management of affected families."
   2. **Group 2–** "Tests for hereditary syndromes with a high probability of linkage to known cancer susceptibility genes, and for which the medical benefit of the identification of a heterozygote ("carrier") is presumed but not established. The potential clinical value and reliability of the test is based on research studies."
   3. **Group 3–** "Tests for individuals without a family history of cancer, in which the significance of the detection of a mutation is not clear; or tests for hereditary syndromes for which germline mutations have been identified only in a small number of families, or for which the medical benefit of the identification of a heterozygote ("carrier") is not established."

X.   **Benefits, Risks, and Limitations of Genetic Testing for Cancer Predisposition**
   A. Not all mutations are detectable by any single laboratory method.
   B. Figure 3.3 delineates the benefits, risks, and limitations of genetic testing for cancer susceptibility.

FIGURE 3.3   Benefits, Limitations, and Risks of Genetic Testing

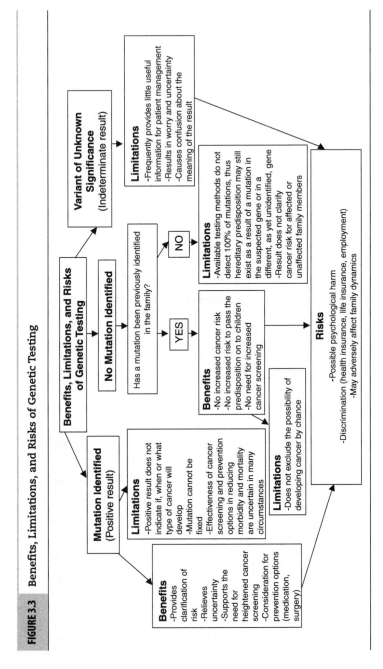

References

1. Gail MH, et al. Projecting individualized probabilities of developing breast cancer for white females who are being examined annually. *J Natl Cancer Inst* 1989;81:1879–1886.

2. Claus EB, Risch N, Thompson WD. Autosomal dominant inheritance of early-onset breast cancer. Implications for risk prediction. *Cancer* 1994;73:643–651.

3. Ford D, et al. Genetic heterogeneity and penetrance analysis of the BRCA1 and BRCA2 genes in breast cancer families. The Breast Cancer Linkage Consortium. *Am J Hum Genet* 1998;62:676–689.

4. Ford D, Easton DF, Peto J. Estimates of the gene frequency of BRCA1 and its contribution to breast and ovarian cancer incidence. *Am J Hum Genet* 1995;57:1457–1462.

5. Claus EB, Risch N, Thompson WD. Genetic analysis of breast cancer in the cancer and steroid hormone study. *Am J Hum Genet* 1991;48:232–242.

6. Miki Y, et al. A strong candidate for the breast and ovarian cancer suscepti-bility gene BRCA1. *Science* 1994;266:66–71.

7. Holt JT, et al. Growth retardation and tumour inhibition by BRCA1. [see comments]. [erratum appears in *Nat Genet* 1998;19:102]. *Nat Genet* 1996;12:298–302.

8. Gayther SA, et al. Germline mutations of the BRCA1 gene in breast and ovarian cancer families provide evidence for a genotype-phenotype correlation. *Nat Genet* 1995;11:428–433.

9. Wu LC, et al. Identification of a RING protein that can interact in vivo with the BRCA1 gene product. *Nat Genet* 1996;14:430–440.

10. Crook T, et al. p53 mutations in BRCA1-associated familial breast cancer. [see comments]. *Lancet* 1997;350:638–639.

11. Scully R, et al. Association of BRCA1 with RAD51 in mitotic and meitotic cells. *Cell* 1997;88:265–275.

12. Tavtigian SV, et al. The complete BRCA2 gene and mutations in chromosome 13q-linked kindreds. *Nat Genet* 1996;12:333–337.

13. Gayther SA, et al. Variation of risks of breast and ovarian cancer associated with different germline mutations of the BRCA2 gene. *Nat Genet* 1997;15:103–105.

14. Sharan SK, et al. Embryonic lethality and radiation hypersensitivity mediated by Rad51 in mice lacking BRCA2. [see comments]. *Nature* 1997;386:804–810.

15. Tonin P, et al. Frequency of recurrent BRCA1 and BRCA2 mutations in Ashkenazi Jewish breast cancer families. *Nat Med* 1996;2:1179–1183.

16. Pathology of familial breast cancer: differences between breast cancers in carriers of BRCA1 or BRCA2 mutations and sporadic cases. Breast Cancer Linkage Consortium. *Lancet* 1997;349:1505–1510.

17. Lakhani SR, et al. Multifactorial analysis of differences between sporadic breast cancers and cancers involving BRCA1 and BRCA2 mutations. [see comments]. *J Natl Cancer Inst* 1998;90:1138–1145.

18. Verhoog LC, et al. Survival and tumour characteristics of breast-cancer patients with germline mutations of BRCA1. *Lancet* 1998;351:316–321.

19. Robson M. Are BRCA1- and BRCA2-associated breast cancers different? Prognosis of BRCA1-associated breast cancer. *J Clin Oncol* 2000;18(suppl):113S–118S.

20. Verhoog LC, et al. Prognostic significance of germline BRCA2 mutations in hereditary breast cancer patients. *J Clin Oncol* 2000;18(suppl):119S–124S.

21. Porter DE, et al. Breast cancer incidence, penetrance and survival in probable carriers of BRCA1 gene mutation in families linked to BRCA1 on chromosome 17q12-21. *Brit J Surg* 1994;81:1512–1515.

22. Marcus JN, et al. Hereditary breast cancer: pathobiology, prognosis, and BRCA1 and BRCA2 gene linkage. *Cancer* 1996;77:697–709.

23. Foulkes WD, et al. Primary node negative breast cancer in BRCA1 mutation carriers has a poor outcome. *Ann Oncol* 2000;11:307–313.

24. Pierce LJ, et al. Effect of radiotherapy after breast-conserving treatment in women with breast cancer and germline BRCA1/2 mutations. *J Clin Oncol* 2000;18:3360–3369.

25. Robson M, et al. Breast conservation therapy for invasive breast cancer in Ashkenazi women with BRCA gene founder mutations. *J Natl Cancer Inst* 1999;91:2112–2117.

26. Stoppa-Lyonnet D, et al. Familial invasive breast cancers: worse outcome related to BRCA1 mutations. *J Clin Oncol* 2000;18:4053–4059.

27. Lee JS, et al. Survival after breast cancer in Ashkenazi Jewish BRCA1 and BRCA2 mutation carriers. *J Natl Cancer Inst* 1999;91:259–263.

28. Gaffney DK, et al. Response to radiation therapy and prognosis in breast cancer patients with BRCA1 and BRCA2 mutations. *Radiother Oncol* 1998;47:129–136.

29. Verhoog LC, et al. Survival in hereditary breast cancer associated with germline mutations of BRCA2. [see comments]. *J Clin Oncol* 1999;17:3396–3402.

30. Sigurdsson H, Agnarsson BA, Jonasson J. Worse survival among breast cancer patients in families carrying the BRCA2 susceptibility gene. *Breast Cancer Res Treat* 1996;37(suppl):33.

31. Loman N, et al. Prognosis and clinical presentation of BRCA2-associated breast cancer. *Eur J Cancer* 2000;36:1365–1373.

32. Nelen M, Padberg GW, Peeters EA, et al. Localization of the gene for Cowden disease to chromosome 10q22-23. *Nat Genet* 1996;13:114–116.

33. Lynch E, Ostermeyer EA, Lee MK, et al. Inherited mutations in PTEN that are associated with breast cancer, cowden disease, and juvenile polyposis. *Am J Hum Genet* 1997;61:1254–1260.

34. Eng C. Will the real Cowden syndrome please stand up: revised diagnostic criteria. *J Med Genet* 2000;37:828–830.

35. Malkin D, Li FP, Strong LC, et al. Germ line p53 mutations in a familial syndrome of breast cancer, sarcomas, and other neoplasms. *Science* 1990;250:1233–1238.

36. Evans S, Mims B, McMasters KM, et al. Exclusion of a p53 germline mutation in a classic Li-Fraumeni syndrome family. *Hum Genet* 1998;102:681–686.

37. Levine A. p53, the cellular gatekeeper for growth and division. *Cell.* 1997;88:323–331.

38. Li F, Fraumeni JF Jr. Soft-tissue sarcomas, breast cancer, and other neoplasms. A familial syndrome? *Ann Intern Med* 1969;71:747–752.

39. Garber J, Goldstein AM, Kantor AF, Dreyfus MG, Fraumeni JF Jr, Li FP. Follow-up study of twenty-four families with Li-Fraumeni syndrome. *Cancer Res* 1991;51:6094–6097.

40. Birch J, Hartley AL, Tricker KJ, et al. Prevalence and diversity of constitutional mutations in the p53 gene among 21 Li-Fraumeni families. *Cancer Res* 1994;54:1298–1304.

41. Sidransky D, Tokino T, Helzlsouer K, et al. Inherited p53 gene mutations in breast cancer. *Cancer Res* 1992;52:2984–2986.

42. Birch J, Blair V, Kelsey AM, et al. Cancer phenotype correlates with constitutional TP53 genotype in families with the Li-Fraumeni syndrome. *Oncogene* 1998;17:1061–1068.

43. Kleihues P, et al. Tumors associated with p53 germline mutations: a synopsis of 91 families. *Am J Pathol* 1997;150:1–13.

44. Hisada M, et al. Multiple primary cancers in families with Li-Fraumeni syndrome. *J Natl Cancer Inst* 1998;90:606–611.

45. Varley JM, et al. Germ-line mutations of TP53 in Li-Fraumeni families: an extended study of 39 families. *Cancer Res* 1997;57:3245–3252.

46. Varley J, Evans DGR, Birch JM. Li-Fraumeni syndrome - a molecular and clinical review. *Br J Cancer* 1997;76:1–14.

47. FitzGerald M, Bean JM, Hegde SR, et al. Heterozygous ATM mutations do not contribute to early onset of breast cancer. *Nat Genet* 1997;15:307–310.

48. Swift M, Reitnauer PJ, Morrell D, Chase CL. Breast and other cancers in families with Ataxia-Telangiectasia. *N Engl J Med* 1987;316:1289–1294.

49. Foroud T, Wei S, Ziv Y, et al. Localization of an ataxia-telangiectasia locus to a 3-cM interval on chromosome 11q23: linkage analysis of 111 families by an international consortium. *Am J Hum Genet* 1991;49:1263–1279.

50. Stavitsky K, Sfez S, Tagle DA, et al. The complete sequence of the coding region of the ATM gene reveals similarity to cell cycle regulators in different species. *Hum Molec Genet* 1995;4:2025–2032.

51. Izatt L, Greenman J, Hodgson S, et al. Identification of germline missense mutations and rare allelic variants in the ATM gene in early-onset breast cancer. *Genes Chrom Cancer* 1999;26:286–294.

52. West C, Elyan SA, Berry P, Cowan R, Scott D. A comparison of the radiosensitivity of lymphocytes from normal donors, cancer patients, individuals with ataxia-telangiectasia (A-T) and A-T heterozygotes. *Intl J Radiat Biol* 1995;68:197–203.

53. Swift M, Morrell D, Massey DB, Chase CL. Incidence of cancer in families affected by ataxia-telangiectasia. *N Engl J Med* 1991;325:1831–1836.

54. Inskip H, Kinlen LJ, Taylor AM, Woods CG, Arlett CF. Risk of breast cancer and other cancers in heterozygotes for ataxia-telangiectasia. *Br J Cancer* 1999;79:1304–1307.

55. Janin N, Andrieu N, Ossian K, Lauge A, Croquette MF, Griselli C., et al. Breast cancer risk in ataxia-telangiectasia (AT) heterozygotes: haplotype study in French AT families. *Br J Cancer* 1999;80:1042–1045.

56. Olsen J, Hahnemann HM, Borresen-Dale AL, et al. Cancer in patients with ataxia-telangiectasia and in their relatives in the Nordic countries. *J Natl Cancer Inst* 2001;93:121–127.

57. Finan M, Ray MK. Gastrointestinal polyposis syndromes. *Dermatol Clin* 1989;7:419–434.

58. Vasen H. Clinical diagnosis and management of hereditary colorectal cancer syndromes. *J Clin Oncol* 2000;18(suppl):81S–92S.

59. Jenne D, Reimann H, Nezu J, Friedel W, Loff S, Muller O, et al. Peutz-Jehgers syndrome is caused by mutations in a novel serine threonine kinase. *Nat Genet* 1997;18:38–43.

60. Hamminiki A, Tomlinson I, Markie D, Jarvinen H, Sistonen P, Bjorkqvist AM, et al. Localization of a susceptibility marker for Peutz-Jehgers syndrome to 19p using comparative genomic hybridization and targeted linkage analysis. *Nat Genet* 1997;15:87–90.

61. Gruber SBE, Entius MM., Petersen GM, et al. Pathogenesis of adenocarcinoma in Peutz-Jeghers syndrome. *Cancer Res* 1998;58:5267–5270.

62. Boardman L, Thibodeau SN, Schaid DJ, et al. Increased risk for cancer in Peutz-Jeghers syndrome. *Ann Intern Med* 1998;128: 896–899.

63. Giardiello FM, et al. Increased risk of cancer in the Peutz-Jeghers syndrome. *N Engl J Med* 1987;316:1511–1514.

64. Wang Z-J, Churchman M, Avizienyte E, et al. Germline mutations of the LKB1 (STK11) gene in Peutz-Jeghers patients. *J Med Genet* 1999;36:365–368.

65. Yilkorkala A, Avizienyte E, Tomlinson IPM, et al. Mutations and impaired function of LKB1 in familial and non-familial Peutz-Jeghers syndrome and a sporadic testicular cancer. *Hum Molec Genet* 1999;8: 45–51.

66. Anonymous. Statement of the American Society of Clinical Oncology: genetic testing for cancer susceptibility, Adopted on February 20, 1996. *J Clin Oncol* 1996;14:1730–1736.

Development of a Risk Assessment Clinic

chapter 4

Vicky Mizell, MS, RN, FNP, CS
Clinical Administrative Director
Cancer Prevention Center
The University of Texas M. D. Anderson Cancer Center
Houston, TX

Therese Bevers, MD
Medical Director
Cancer Prevention Center
The University of Texas M. D. Anderson Cancer Center
Houston, TX

I.   **The Emergence of Risk Assessment Clinics**
   A. Risk assessment clinics emerged due to advances in cancer genetics.
      1. *Advances in cancer genetics and identification of risk factors have significantly increased the challenges and opportunities to provide comprehensive cancer risk evaluation and counseling. Scientific advances have identified a growing number of risk factors that predispose to cancer. Recent research related to breast cancer prevention has highlighted the need for cancer risk assessment.*
      2. *Risk assessment programs have gained popularity as early detection continues to improve clinical outcomes.*
   B. Media attention to the familial or hereditary component of some cancers has increased public awareness and demand for better identification of individuals at risk as well as prevention.
   C. Knowledge deficit and misunderstanding of indications for genetic testing, pretest counseling, signature of consent forms, and interpretation of genetic test results among general practice physicians highlights the need for specialized clinics to address cancer risk assessment.[1,2]
   D. Many health-care centers have created programs to identify high-risk individuals by developing risk assessment clinics. These clinics provide a centralized location for identifying personal risk factors that are used to design personalized early detection and prevention strategies. Some risk assessment clinics offer genetic testing to patients whose family histories suggest hereditary predisposition to cancer. However, genetic testing should be considered as a tool in risk assessment rather than as an end in itself. A more important goal is to establish a program to identify individuals at increased risk, to educate and counsel them, and to facilitate appropriate management and screening measures.[5]
   E. Risk assessment clinics should provide universal appropriate screening and standardization of screening methodology.
   F. Recommendations might include prophylactic surgery, chemoprevention, or earlier or more frequent cancer screening.

II. **Cancer Risk Assessment Services Are Delivered in a Broad Range of Clinical Settings.[3]**
   A. Research/academic setting
      1. *A multidisciplinary subspecialty clinic for cancer risk assessment services is provided.*
      2. *Thorough pretest and posttest counseling is provided.*
      3. *There are well-defined eligibility criteria.*
      4. *IRB-approved protocols are often followed.*
      5. *There is a mechanism for tracking outcomes.*
      6. *Members of staff are often cross-trained in oncology and cancer genetics.*
      7. *Most major centers are directed by a board-certified oncologist with focused training in cancer genetics.*
      8. *Other centers use a board-certified clinician such as a clinical molecular geneticist.*

9. *Additional members of the team may include certified genetic counselors with cancer genetics experience or advanced practice nurses with masters-level training in genetics and oncology experience in primary counseling roles.*

10. *Other support staff may include clinical social workers and mental health professionals.*

B. Private/clinical

1. *Ordering genetic testing is no longer restricted to research settings.*

2. *Private clinicians may order commercial analysis of several cancer-associated genes for patients.*

3. *A significant potential exists for misinterpretation of results by clinicians and misinformation for patients.*[1,3]

4. *Most private physicians who finished training before the late 1990s have not had any hands-on experience with ordering or interpreting cancer genetic tests.*

5. *Pretest and posttest counseling and informed consent guidelines are published by commercial genetic testing vendors. However, the vendor cannot ensure that these measures are done in the private/clinical model.*

6. *Risk assessment and genetic testing offered by a private physician can be rewarding due to the established patient-physician relationship. However, potential lack of third-party reimbursement and time constraints are limiting factors.*

III. **Benefits/Advantages of Risk Assessment** [3,4]

A. Those who benefit are those who might otherwise have died from their disease without risk assessment.

B. There is reassurance for those with negative test results.

C. Less radical treatment may be needed to cure patients.

D. There is a lower treatment cost if less radical treatment is required.

E. Risk assessment programs differentiate cancer programs by demonstrating commitment to patient services along the full continuum of care, thereby enhancing brand recognition within the community.

F. Risk assessment programs may increase screening compliance rates by sending periodic reminders to individuals assessed at the clinic.

G. Risk assessment programs provide an ideal forum for identifying and counseling persons who may be eligible for clinical trials.

H. Risk assessment programs may provide a platform for translating advances in genetic research into clinical practice. Given the widespread media attention on genetic research, it is likely that more patients will seek out these services in the future. Programs that offer risk assessment services will be well positioned to respond to patients' growing appetite for risk evaluation strategies, as well as to physicians' increasing needs for support in this area.

IV.   **Defining a Risk Assessment Program**[5]

    A.   The primary goal of a risk assessment program should be to provide effective, efficient comprehensive risk assessment services to individuals at high risk for developing cancer.

    B.   A risk assessment clinic may serve as a link to well populations relevant to research initiatives, or it can be an effective health promotion and outreach activity.

    C.   A risk assessment clinic may be used as a public relations vehicle for the sponsoring institution.

    D.   The mission of a risk assessment clinic should be clearly defined. Programs that wish to serve the broad population, not just marketing and outreach efforts to physicians, should publicize their service to the public at large.

    E.   Risk assessment clinics can provide the following services:

        1.   *Assessment and evaluation of cancer risk*

        2.   *Screening services*

        3.   *Genetic testing*

        4.   *Counseling services*

        5.   *Patient education*

        6.   *Focal point for cancer genetics education for an entire health-care network*

        7.   *Serve as a resource for the development of relevant guidelines and standards*

        8.   *Serve as a repository of information to help track data*

        9.   *Serve as a consultation resource for clinicians, centralizing the effort to identify high-risk individuals*

        10.   *Manage high-risk patients in a more cost-efficient and time-efficient manner*

V.   **Developing a Risk Assessment Clinic**

    A.   The first step is to develop a mission statement and identify objectives.

    B.   Clearly delineate the scope of the clinic services including target population.[5]

        1.   *Determine if services will be limited to a single cancer type or multiple hereditary cancer syndromes.*

            a.   The scope of services will be somewhat determined by the expertise and interest of the staff and the availability of expert consultation.

        2.   *Identify types of individuals who will be candidates for risk assessment.*

        3.   *Clarify what components of cancer risk counseling will be offered. Will the services be consultative or comprehensive?*

        4.   *Will genetic testing be included as part of the comprehensive services?*

    C.   Determine eligibility criteria for individuals to receive risk assessment services.[5]

        1.   *Individuals with a strong family history of cancer*

        2.   *Individuals who perceive themselves to be at increased risk*

3. Individuals without factors suggesting a genetic predisposition who have had a biopsy diagnosis of atypical hyperplasia or lobular carcinoma in situ

4. Individuals desiring risk reduction strategies, for example, prophylactic mastectomy and chemoprevention

VI. **Key Elements of a Risk Assessment Clinic**[1]

A. Multidisciplinary consultation team

1. Expertise in cancer etiology, screening, diagnosis, and treatment.

2. Expertise in basic genetics and cancer genetics.

3. Skills related to cancer experience and fear of the disease.

4. Multidisciplinary team with skills in genetics, nursing, and mental health.

5. The team should include a physician (medical, surgical, radiation, or gynecology oncologist or clinical geneticist). Other team members may include an advanced practice oncology nurse, registered nurses, genetic counselors, mental health professionals, and health educators.[6]

6. Several staffing models have been recommended which use different disciplines to address the different areas of a risk assessment clinic.[5] Cancer expertise can be provided by a physician, nurse, or nurse practitioner. Genetic expertise can be addressed by a genetics counselor, physician, nurse, or nurse practitioner. Counseling can be addressed by a psychologist, genetics counselor, nurse, physician, or social worker. The physical examination should be provided by a physician or nurse practitioner.[6] Scheduling can be provided by clerical staff. Members of the team will require initial and frequent education and training (Table 4.1).

B. Space allocation

1. The risk assessment clinic should be located proximal to associated screening services and accessible to the multidisciplinary staff.

2. The rooms should be esthetically pleasing, comfortable for lengthy discussion, and large enough to accommodate several family members.[7]

3. Office space should be allocated for administrative and clerical staff, computers, printers, fax machines, telephones, reference library, and centralized locked file cabinets.

TABLE 4.1	**Educational Resources for Genetic Cancer Risk Assessment**

- American Cancer Society (ACS)
- American Society of Clinical Oncologists (ASCO)
- National Society of Genetics Counselors (NSGC)
- Oncology Nursing Society (ONS)
- International Society of Nurses in Genetics (ISONG)
- National Coalition for Health Professional Education in Genetics

    4. *The lobby with receptionist should be separate from cancer patients, if at all possible.*

    5. *Consider sharing space with other clinical programs to offset costs.*

C. Scheduling

    1. *Prior to scheduling, determine availability of staff, space allocation, number of visits, and length of each visit.*

    2. *A survey of cancer centers revealed a range from one to three visits per patient and an average total consultation time of 129 minutes.[8]*

    3. *Consider scheduling the appointment only after the patient has returned a family history questionnaire and obtained all available documentation of family medical history, so that the session can be focused on counseling.[5]*

D. Comprehensive assessment tool

    1. *A risk profile is derived from a family history questionnaire, personal medical history (e.g., previous biopsy), lifestyle behaviors, and (in some cases) genetic testing.*

    2. *Statistical models (e.g., Gail, Claus, BRCAPRO) can be used to quantify risk evaluations and complement qualitative assessments (see the National Cancer Institute web site at http://bcra.nci.nih.gov/brc/).*

E. Cancer risk counseling process

    1. *The goal is to increase the individual's awareness of their cancer risk.*

    2. *Counseling should emphasize the benefit of risk reduction strategies and early detection while minimizing anxiety that might reduce compliance with screening exams.*

    3. *The risk assessment team should assess the patient's reason for seeking counseling. Understanding the patient's agenda will help the staff individualize the content of the patient counseling interaction.*

    4. *The risk assessment team should assess the patient's beliefs and understanding about cancer.*

    5. *The risk assessment team should assess the patient's level of anxiety and coping skills.*

    6. *The family health questionnaire is used to construct a pedigree.*

    7. *Familial cancer risk is determined by the pedigree.*

    8. *Communicating risk information is facilitated as follows:*

        a. The risk assessment team should assess the individual's preconceived estimation of their cancer risk.

        b. Frame information in a positive manner, being sensitive and maintaining the strictest confidence.

    9. *The risk assessment team provides recommendations for screening and risk reduction.*

    10. *Counseling is provided for managing the risk of developing cancer.*

F. Genetic testing[5]

   1. *Risk assessment clinics should be able to offer genetic testing to high-risk individuals or be able to make appropriate referrals for testing.*

   2. *Genetic testing should begin with a living family member with cancer.*

   3. *Risk assessment clinics that offer genetic testing must provide adequate education of staff, allow for pretest and posttest counseling, and procedures for maintaining confidentiality and providing for informed consent.*

   4. *The risk and benefits of genetic testing must be thoroughly discussed with the patient.*

   5. *Genetic testing does not provide a diagnosis but a probability for developing cancer.*

   6. *Recommendations for management of risk assessment and genetic testing must be standardized with guidelines that can be followed by all staff members.*

G. Follow-up surveillance plan

   1. *All participants receive risk reduction and screening recommendations tailored to their individual risk profile.*

   2. *All participants are presented with the option to return to the clinic for reevaluation.*

      a. If personal history or personal medical history change

      b. Additional counseling provided as necessary

H. Post-assessment summary

   1. *All participants receive a detailed letter reinforcing basic education, personal cancer risk reduction, and screening recommendations.*

   2. *If patient desires, referring physicians also receive documentation of visit results so that they may ensure appropriate follow-up and enhance risk factor identification skills.*

I. Confidentiality assurance

   1. *Separate records should be maintained to protect against possible social, employment, or insurance discrimination.*

   2. *General results of risk assessment are shared with referring physician, if desired by the patient. Genetic testing information may be included in a letter to the referring physician depending on patient preference.*

J. Marketing strategies

   1. *Institutional web site*

      a. Link to on-line risk assessment questionnaire

      b. Advertising campaign

         i. Brochures distributed to family practice physicians and oncologists

   2. *Off-site lectures/presentations*

   3. *Publications*

K. Data management systems
   1. *Risk assessment clinic needs an adequate system to manage:*
      a. Telephone consultation
      b. Registering patients
      c. Scheduling patients
      d. Developing pedigree from family history questionnaire
      e. Clinical records
      f. Results reporting
      g. Clinical outcomes
      h. Quality assurance
      i. Billing
      j. Financial reporting

VII. Reimbursement
  A. Risk counseling services are rarely covered by third-party insurance.
  B. Genetic testing may be a covered benefit. However, a patient may not desire that an insurance company to be aware of genetic testing.

VIII. Challenges to a Risk Assessment Clinic[9]
  A. Development of community referral patterns
    1. *Essential to keep community physicians apprised of patient's progress during risk consultation*
    2. *Establish referral policies[10]*
  B. Development of system for assigning patients into discrete risk categories
  C. Reimbursement of risk assessment services
    1. *View risk assessment as a service enhancement to patients and referring physicians rather than as a significant source of revenues.*
    2. *Risk counseling is not usually covered by third-party payers.*

IX. Patient Intake Phase (Figure 4.1)
  A. Individuals contact the Cancer Prevention Center at The University of Texas M. D. Anderson Cancer Center requesting risk counseling. The secretary triages the call (Figures 4.1 and 4.2).
  B. A Family History Questionnaire is mailed to individuals who are determined to be at increased risk according to the telephone triage criteria. A stamped, addressed envelope to the Cancer Prevention Center Genetic Counselor is enclosed for the patient's convenience. The Risk Assessment Program at The University of Texas M. D. Anderson Cancer Center was started in 1996. Approximately 20 to 30 % of patients seen are found to be of low or moderate risk for cancer development.
  C. When the Family History Questionnaire is received in the Cancer Prevention Center, the secretary logs the questionnaire into the Risk Assessment Database. The date the questionnaire was received along with the individual's name is entered (Figure 4.3).

FIGURE 4.1 Flow Diagram for Risk Assessment Clinic
The University of Texas M.D. Anderson Cancer Center
Cancer Prevention Center

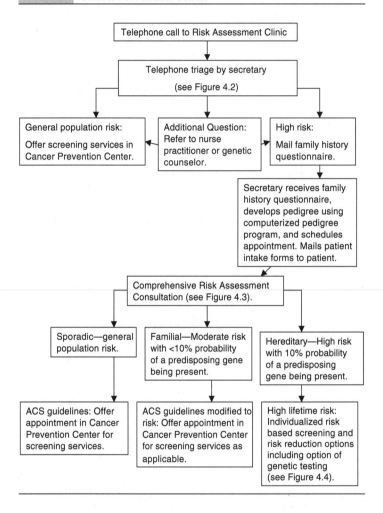

D. The secretary determines if the individual is already a patient at The University of Texas M. D. Anderson Cancer Center.

E. The secretary contacts the individual by telephone to obtain demographic and insurance information from all new patients.

F. The secretary schedules a risk assessment appointment for the patient.

FIGURE 4.2	Telephone Triage for Callers Without Cancer The University of Texas M.D. Anderson Cancer Center Cancer Prevention Center

1. Are there two family members that have breast cancer, ovarian cancer, or one with each type of cancer?

No   Yes

Mail questionnaire (and have them return to the Cancer Prevention Center).

2. Is there a family member who has both a breast cancer and an ovarian cancer?

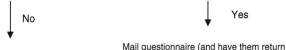

No   Yes

Mail questionnaire (and have them return to the Cancer Prevention Center).

3. Are there any family members with a breast cancer or an ovarian cancer diagnosed before the age of 40?

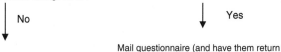

No   Yes

Mail questionnaire (and have them return to the Cancer Prevention Center).

4. Are you of Ashkenazi Jewish origin and have one family member with a breast cancer or an ovarian cancer?

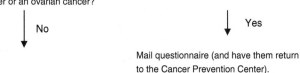

No   Yes

Mail questionnaire (and have them return to the Cancer Prevention Center).

5. Are there any males in your family with breast cancer?

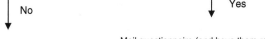

No   Yes

Mail questionnaire (and have them return to the Cancer Prevention Center).

Secretary script:

Thank you for your interest in the risk assessment clinic. The answers to these questions tell us that you have no family history for breast or ovarian cancer that would suggest an inherited risk for one of these cancers. If you still feel that you would like to come to the clinic for risk evaluation, we will mail a questionnaire and have someone give you a call after you return it to M.D. Anderson to schedule a risk counseling appointment.

FIGURE 4.3   Comprehensive Risk Assessment Consultation
The University of Texas M.D. Anderson Cancer Center
Cancer Prevention Center

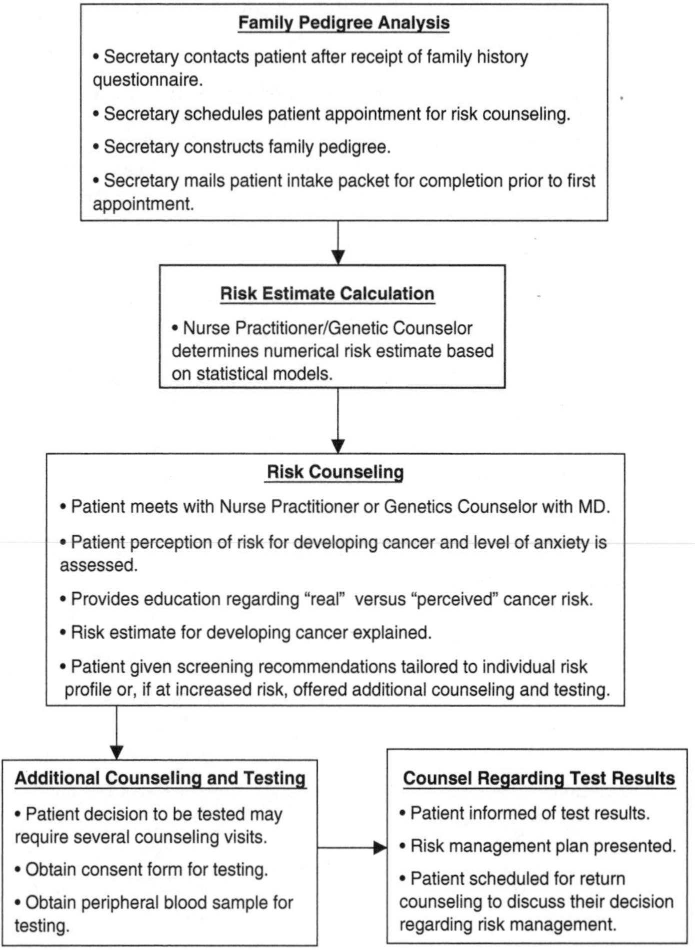

Family Pedigree Analysis

• Secretary contacts patient after receipt of family history questionnaire.

• Secretary schedules patient appointment for risk counseling.

• Secretary constructs family pedigree.

• Secretary mails patient intake packet for completion prior to first appointment.

Risk Estimate Calculation

• Nurse Practitioner/Genetic Counselor determines numerical risk estimate based on statistical models.

Risk Counseling

• Patient meets with Nurse Practitioner or Genetics Counselor with MD.

• Patient perception of risk for developing cancer and level of anxiety is assessed.

• Provides education regarding "real" versus "perceived" cancer risk.

• Risk estimate for developing cancer explained.

• Patient given screening recommendations tailored to individual risk profile or, if at increased risk, offered additional counseling and testing.

Additional Counseling and Testing

• Patient decision to be tested may require several counseling visits.

• Obtain consent form for testing.

• Obtain peripheral blood sample for testing.

Counsel Regarding Test Results

• Patient informed of test results.

• Risk management plan presented.

• Patient scheduled for return counseling to discuss their decision regarding risk management.

G. The secretary reserves a counseling room for the date and time of the appointment.

H. The secretary prepares the pedigree according to the Family History Questionnaire.

I. The secretary assembles a patient folder for new patients.

    J. An intake package is mailed to the patient confirming their appointment, including directions to the clinic with parking information and forms to complete and bring to the appointment.

    K. The patient folder is submitted to the risk assessment team one week prior to the scheduled appointment for their review and preparation of information regarding their individual breast cancer risk.

X.   **Comprehensive Risk Consultation (Figure 4.3, Table 4.2)**

    A. The patient arrives for risk assessment counseling appointment with genetic counselor and physician.

    B. The genetics counselor and physician or the nurse practitioner review the Family Pedigree Analysis and inform the patient of their risk estimate.

    C. Individuals with general population risk or familial moderate risk with <10% probability of a predisposing gene being present are offered an appointment in the Cancer Prevention Center for cancer screening services which follow the American Cancer Society (ACS) guidelines (Figure 4.1).

    D. Individuals with a high lifetime risk are provided risk-based screening and risk reduction options including the option of DNA testing (Figure 4.4).

TABLE 4.2   Comprehensive Risk Consultation
The University of Texas M. D. Anderson Cancer Center
Cancer Prevention Center

Comprehensive Risk Consultation

Phase	Process
1. Family pedigree analysis	• Review pedigree with patient
2. Risk factor education	• Provide basic education regarding "real" versus "perceived" cancer risk
	• Explain concept of cancer genetics
3. Risk estimate calculation	• Calculate numerical risk estimate based on statistical models as well as clinical experience
4. Screening recommendation	• Offer screening recommendations including genetic testing tailored to individual risk profile
	• Recommendation for follow-up screening
5. Summary letter	• Patient receives detailed letter summarizing risk assessment process, genetic testing, and screening recommendations.
	• If patient desires, referring physician receives similar letter explaining consultative process and recommendations.

E. Patients who accept DNA testing are scheduled for a follow-up appointment with the nurse practitioner or genetic counselor, at which time the patient signs an informed consent, receives additional genetic counseling, and a peripheral blood sample for genetic testing is obtained. A follow-up appointment is scheduled to review DNA test results. If genetic mutations are found, management options are discussed with the patient. Testing and genetic counseling are offered to other interested family members. If no genetic mutations are found, an individualized screening recommendation based on risk is provided (Figure 4.4).

FIGURE 4.4   **Genetic Testing**
The University of Texas M.D. Anderson Cancer Center Cancer Prevention Center

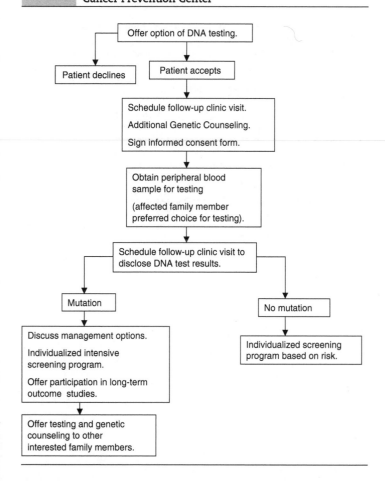

    F. The comprehensive risk consultation is followed with a summary letter sent to both the patient and referring physician (if applicable).

XI. Conclusion

A. With increasing modalities of breast cancer risk reduction and risk-based screening recommendations, it is critical that women fully understand their breast cancer risk and which options are appropriate, based on their risk.

References

1. Giardiello FM, Brensinger JD, Peterson GM, Luce MC, Hylind LM, et al. The use and interpretation of commercial APC gene testing for familial adenomatous polyposis. *N Engl J Med* 1997;336: 823–827.

2. Rowley PT, Loader S. Attitudes of obstetrician-gynecologists toward DNA testing for a genetic susceptibility to breast cancer. *Obstetr Gynecol* 1996;88:611–615.

3. Weitzel JN. Genetic cancer risk assessment. Putting it all together. *Cancer* 1999;86(11 Suppl):2483–2492.

4. Weitzel JN. Genetic counseling for familial cancer risk. *Hosp Pract* 1996;31:57–69.

5. Roche CA, Lucas MR, Hughes KS. Development of a risk assessment clinic. In: Vogel VG, ed. *Management of Patients at High Risk for Breast Cancer.* Malden, MA: Blackwell Science, Inc; 2001:166–182.

6. Kelly PT. Cancer risk information services: promise and pitfalls. *Breast J* 1996;2:233–237.

7. Peters JA. Familial cancer risk: impact on today's oncology practice. *J Oncol Mgt* September–October 1994:20–30.

8. Thompson JA, Wiesner GL, Sellers T, et al. Genetic services for familial cancer patients: a survey of national cancer institute cancer centers. *J Natl Cancer Inst* 1995;87:1446–1455.

9. The Oncology Roundtable. Cancer risk assessment clinics. Managing the needs of the "worried well." *Clin Watch;* 1999; 17:1–14.

10. Reintgen DS, Clark RA. Operational issues in developing a cancer screening program. *Cancer Screening* 1996; 277–289.

Breast Imaging

Lara A. Hardesty, MD
Assistant Professor of Radiology
Magee Womens Hospital
University of Pittsburgh School of Medicine

chapter 5

I.   **Mammography**

   A. Mammography is the foundation of breast imaging. Mammography is used to screen asymptomatic women for breast cancer and is the basis for the imaging evaluation of breast symptoms.

   B. Types of Mammography

     1. *Screening Mammography*

       a. Screen asymptomatic women for breast cancer.

       b. Mortality from breast cancer can be reduced by 30%.[1]

       c. Mammography is very sensitive for detection of an abnormality, with sensitivity of 85 to 90% [2], but not very specific. Only 30% of mammographically detected lesions that are biopsied are malignant.[2]

       d. Age guidelines

         i. Mammography is recommended yearly beginning at age 40.

         ii. No official guidelines have been published regarding upper age limit.

         iii. No guidelines have been published regarding screening of "high risk" women. Our institution's recommendation is to screen women whose mother or sister developed breast cancer before age 50 at yearly screening intervals beginning 10 years younger than the age at which their relative was diagnosed with breast cancer. If their relative was diagnosed at age 50 or older, then routine screening recommendations (annually after age 40) are appropriate.

     2. *Diagnostic Mammography*

       a. Evaluate symptomatic women, including those with:

         i. Palpable lump

         ii. Nipple discharge

         iii. Breast pain (acute onset)

         iv. History of breast cancer

         v. History of biopsy proven benign breast disease

         vi. Breast implants

         vii. Follow-up of previously seen mammographic lesion (as directed by radiologist on report from prior mammogram)

         viii. Axillary adenopathy

         ix. Metastasis of unknown primary

         x. Change in size, shape, or color of breast, nipple, or skin

   C. Mammography Technique

     1. *Standard mammography includes two views of each breast being evaluated. The view from superior-to-inferior plane is called the cranial-caudal (CC) projection. The view from medial-to-lateral plane is called the medial-lateral-oblique (MLO) projection.*

     2. *Screening mammography includes a cranial-caudal (CC) view of each breast and a medial-lateral-oblique (MLO) view of each breast.*

     3. *Diagnostic mammography includes a cranial-caudal (CC) view of each breast being evaluated, a medial-lateral-oblique (MLO) view, and a true lateral view of each breast being evaluated.*

4. *Once the radiologist reviews the basic mammographic views, the radiologist directs the mammographic technologist to obtain additional "specialized" views that are tailored to the evaluation of that particular patient. Some of the more commonly utilized additional views include:*
   a. Spot compression views to press out the area of concern to discern if a lesion is present or if overlapping glandular tissue is causing an apparent false lesion
   b. Magnification views to enlarge microcalcifications or small nodules to permit better evaluation of their features

D. Mammography Findings
   1. *Nodules/Masses*
      a. The borders of these lesions and their overall shape are evaluated to distinguish benign from malignant.
         i. Round or oval with smooth borders are generally benign and commonly include:
            • Cyst
            • Fibroadenoma—a benign solid tumor
            • Lymph node
         ii. Irregularly marginated lesions are suspicious for breast malignancy.
   2. *Calcifications*
      a. Suspicious for malignancy
         i. Focal clustered
         ii. Pleomorphic in size and shape
         iii. Branching forms
      b. Benign-appearing calcifications
         i. Scattered, especially when bilateral
         ii. Coarse
         iii. Vascular
         iv. Popcorn—a type of coarse calcification that is classic for a degenerating fibroadenoma, a benign solid tumor
         v. Teacupping equals milk of calcium—describes the classic appearance of calcium layering (via gravity) in the bottom of microcysts in fibrocystic process, benign
   3. *Asymmetry*
      a. Describes an asymmetry of density mammographically between one breast and the other in a symmetric area of the breasts
         i. Stable asymmetric glandular density equals benign, common.
         ii. New asymmetry equals possible breast cancer.
   4. *Architectural Distortion*
      a. Describes a pulling-in focally in a breast on mammogram
         i. Stable and at the site of a prior surgical scar equals benign.
         ii. New equals possible breast cancer.

II. **Breast Ultrasound**
   A. Ultrasound is used to obtain additional information about known lesions that have been discovered either on mammogram or on physical examination.[3]

B. Screening ultrasound to evaluate asymptomatic women for breast cancer is not currently the standard of care.

C. Ultrasound determines whether a lesion is:

1. *Cystic (liquid and benign)*
   a. Lesion must meet all three of these criteria:
      i. Round or oval in shape
      ii. Anechoic (black on ultrasound)
      iii. Demonstrates posterior acoustic enhancement

2. *Solid (may be benign or malignant—further evaluation is necessary)*
   a. Lesion is hypoechoic (gray on ultrasound) and may have any shape.

3. *Indeterminate (may be a debris-filled cyst or a solid lesion— further evaluation is necessary to exclude malignancy)*

III. Imaging-Guided Percutaneous Breast Biopsy

A. Indications

1. *To determine whether a visualized suspicious lesion is benign or malignant.*
   a. If the lesion is proven to be benign, surgical excision is not required in the majority of cases.
   b. If the lesion is proven to be malignant at biopsy, knowledge of this preoperatively allows the surgeon to plan a one-step definitive operative procedure to excise the cancer with clean margins and to perform axillary node evaluation.

B. Types of Imaging-Guided Percutaneous Biopsies

1. *Fine Needle Aspiration (FNA) Biopsy*
   a. Uses:
      i. Aspirate known cyst for symptom relief. Fluid is discarded.
      ii. Determine whether a hypoechoic lesion is a complex cyst (benign) or is solid (potentially malignant) and requires microscopic analysis.
      iii. Obtain sample for microscopic analysis when the lesion is smaller than 5 mm in size and thus difficult to target with a core biopsy needle.
   b. Equipment: 19 or 21 gauge needle and plastic tubing and syringe

2. *Core Needle Biopsy*
   a. Spring-Loaded Core Biopsy Needle
      i. 14 gauge is the most commonly used size.
      ii. Obtain solid cores of tissue for microscopic analysis.
         • Requires multiple (3–5) passes with the needle
   b. Vacuum-Assisted Core Biopsy Needle
      i. An 11 gauge or 14 gauge needle is used.
      ii. Marking clips can be placed to mark the site of biopsy at the completion of the procedure (only if 11 gauge needle size is utilized).
      iii. There is a solitary puncture of skin with the needle, and the needle then rotates circumferentially, obtaining core tissue samples at multiple locations. The tissue samples are withdrawn through the bore of the needle while the needle remains within the breast, enabling multiple samples to be obtained with one needle placement.

3. *Types of Imaging Guidance for Needle Biopsies*
   a. Ultrasound Guided[4]
      i. Fine needle aspiration biopsies or core biopsies
   b. Stereotactic (Mammographically) Guided[5,6]
      i. This is used for core biopsies only.
      ii. Two mammographic images obtained at predictable angles allow calculation of the location of breast lesion by computer, permitting the lesion to be targeted for biopsy.

IV. **Needle Localization for Surgical Excision**
   A. Indication: to mark a nonpalpable lesion (detected either on mammography or sonography) for surgical excision.
   B. Using either mammographic or sonographic guidance, the radiologist places a needle into the lesion of concern. Through the bore of this needle, a thin wire is placed to mark the lesion for the surgeon, and the needle is removed, leaving the wire in place to serve as a map for the surgeon intraoperatively.
   C. After surgical excision of the lesion, the tissue specimen is imaged (either radiographically or sonographically) to confirm that the area of concern has been successfully excised.

V. **Sentinel Axillary Node Imaging or Lymphoscintigraphy**
   A. Purpose: a method of evaluating the axillary lymph nodes for metastatic spread of breast cancer. This serves as an alternative to the traditional method of axillary lymph node dissection.
   B. Principle
      1. *The sentinel axillary lymph node is the first node in the axillary lymph node drainage basin into which the lymph from the breast cancer flows. All lymph flowing into the axillary lymph nodes must first pass through the axillary sentinel node. Thus, if there are no metastatic breast cancer cells in the sentinel axillary lymph node, then theoretically none of the axillary lymph nodes will contain metastatic breast cancer cells and traditional axillary dissection can be avoided (decreasing the risk of later lymphedema).*
   C. Techniques: Multiple techniques have been tested and have been shown to be similarly successful. The protocol currently used at our institution is:
      1. *Injection of Radiopharmaceutical*
         a. 0.5 millicuries of Technetium 99m filtered sulfur colloid (0.45 micron size particles) is diluted in 0.3 cc of saline and placed in a tuberculine syringe. This is injected intradermally overlying the tumor site.
      2. *Gamma-Camera Scanning of the Breast and Axilla for Radioactivity*
         a. Performed one hour after injection of the tracer, this produces an image of the activity in the breast (at the site of injection) and in the axillary lymph nodes to serve as a map for the surgeon intraoperatively.
         b. At some institutions, no gamma-camera scanning is performed. The intraoperative handheld probe is felt to be sufficient to guide the surgeon during sentinel node excision.

VI.   **Future Breast Imaging Possibilities**

A. Mammography in combination with sonography is currently the best method for the early detection of breast cancer, but it has limitations. Complementary new techniques with which to image breast cancer include:

1. *Breast Magnetic Resonance Imaging (MRI)*

   a. Technique

      i. MRI detects breast cancers by evaluating two characteristics of a breast lesion, morphology and enhancement.

         • Morphology is analysis of the lesion's shape and borders. Cancers tend to have irregular shapes and poorly defined margins while benign lesions tend to be round or oval shaped with smooth margins.

         • Enhancement of breast carcinomas after the intravenous injection of gadopentetate dimeglumine is prompt relative to the uptake of this agent by benign breast lesions. In addition, the washout of this contrast agent from carcinomas is faster than it is from benign breast lesions. These enhancement characteristics of malignancies are due to the highly vascular nature of breast malignancies relative to that of benign breast lesions.

      ii. Most breast MRI to date has been performed using 1.5 Tesla magnets, those conventionally used to image other body parts.

      iii. A dedicated breast 0.5 Tesla magnet is now available. Hopefully, these units' lower cost and fewer shielding requirements will enable them to be placed directly within breast imaging centers, allowing breast MRI to be more practical. This is the unit that our institution uses.

      iv. Specific MRI protocols vary but involve imaging of the breasts in multiple planes (most commonly sagittal and axial planes) with thin slice thicknesses (3 mm) before and after the intravenous injection of the contrast agent.[7–9]

   b. Potential Uses

      i. To search for mammographically occult multifocal or multicentric breast carcinoma preoperatively in patients with newly diagnosed breast carcinoma who have mammographically dense breasts.

      ii. To identify the size and location of residual carcinoma in the breast after surgical excision biopsy or segmental mastectomy in which the surgical tissue specimen showed carcinoma extending to the surgical margins. This can help the surgeon plan the extent of the required reexcision.

      iii. To search for a mammographically and sonographically occult primary breast malignancy in patients with biopsy proven carcinoma of unknown origin in an axillary lymph node.

      iv. To evaluate silicone breast implants for intracapsular or extracapsular rupture (this use of breast MRI is currently the standard of care).

   c. Current Limitations

      i. Ability to localize a lesion that is suspicious for carcinoma and is identified only on MRI is limited. There is no currently available device to help place the needle into the correct spot. Currently at our institution, the needle placement is done "freehand."

  ii. Once a surgical biopsy specimen is removed from the breast, there is currently no method to image the specimen and ensure that the MRI-suspicious lesion has been removed.

  iii. While sensitivity for breast malignancy is high, 94 to 100%, specificity is variable, reportedly between 37% and 97%.[7,8,10–14] This means that breast MRI has many false-positive lesions that require further imaging evaluation, often requiring needle biopsy, to exclude malignancy.

  iv. MRI's sensitivity for noninvasive breast carcinoma (ductal carcinoma in situ or DCIS) is unknown. DCIS is often indistinguishable from benign proliferative fibrocystic disease.[7]

 d. Future Possibilities

  i. MRI has great promise as an additional problem-solving tool for the diagnosis of breast malignancy, particularly nonpalpable breast malignancies undetectable by conventional breast imaging. Its expense and high incidence of false-positive results require that it be used in carefully chosen patients.

  ii. The potential role it may play in screening patients at high risk of breast malignancy who have dense breasts mammographically remains to be determined.

2. *Position Emission Tomography (PET) Breast Imaging*

 a. Technique

  i. PET uses positron-emitting radionuclides that decay by emitting two photons that travel in opposite directions.

  ii. PET scanners detect these two photons 180 degrees apart, called coincidence detection.

  iii. PET radionuclides have a short half-life and must be manufactured in a cyclotron.

  iv. PET imaging of the breast uses Fluorine-18 (a positron emitter) that has been incorporated into fluorodeoxyglucose (FDG), a structural analog of glucose.

  v. Tumor cells have increased consumption of glucose relative to normal breast tissue cells. This enables detection of breast cancer cells with PET scanning.

 b. Potential Uses

  i. On small-scale research studies, PET scanning has shown the ability to evaluate the breasts, the axillae (for nodal metastases), and the whole body (for distant metastases).

  ii. Proposed future uses for PET in breast cancer imaging include:

    • Noninvasive evaluation of axillary and internal mammary chain lymph nodes

    • Total body staging for metastases

    • Detection of breast cancer in breasts in which mammography is notoriously limited, including extremely dense breasts, postoperative breasts, and breasts containing implants for augmentation

 c. Current Limitations

  i. Size Detection Threshold

    • The resolution of most modern PET scanners is one centimeter, making detection of lesions smaller than one centimeter very difficult.

- The sensitivity of PET in detecting primary breast cancer ranges from 80 to 100%, and specificity ranges from 86 to 100%.[15–21]
- For primary breast tumors one centimeter or larger, the sensitivity of PET is nearly 100%.[15,16]
- The sensitivity of PET for primary breast tumors smaller than one centimeter is unknown.[22,23]
- The sensitivity of PET for detection of sub-centimeter axillary and distant metastases from breast cancer is also unknown.

ii. Cost
- PET scanning is expensive. PET scanners cost between $1 million and $2 million, and access to a cyclotron is needed to produce the positron-emitting radiopharmaceuticals.

iii. Lesion Localization
- If PET scanning identifies a lesion that is not visible on traditional breast imaging modalities, there is currently no method to localize or mark this area for surgical excision.

d. Future Possibilities
   i. If scanner size detection threshold can be improved and the costs reduced, PET scanning may become an important method of imaging breast cancer in the future. Currently, it is being used in the evaluation of difficult cases at several academic breast centers.

3. *Technetium-99m Sestamibi Scintimammography*

a. Technique
   i. 20 millicuries technetium-99m sestamibi IV into arm contralateral to the breast of concern (prevents false-positive study if axillary lymph nodes uptake the tracer if venous extravasation occurs during injection)
   ii. Images include lateral image of each breast (patient prone) and whole chest image with arms raised to depict the axillae (patient supine), imaged at both early (10 minutes) and delayed (60 minutes) after tracer injection
   iii. Image interpretation
      - Normal study equals uniform tracer uptake in the breast.
      - Abnormal study equals hot spot or zone of focally increased uptake at the site concerning for breast cancer.
   iv. Whole body radiation dose is 0.3 rad, and breast radiation dose is similar to that from a total body bone scan.[24]

b. Potential Uses
   i. On small-scale research studies, Tc-99m sestamibi scanning has shown the ability to evaluate the breasts and the axillae (nodal metastases) for breast cancer. Its role is still being investigated.
   ii. Tc-99m sestamibi scanning has been approved by FDA for breast cancer imaging.
   iii. Tc-99m sestamibi scanning will never replace mammography as a screening test for breast cancer.
   iv. Tc-99m sestamibi scanning may become an adjunct to mammography and sonography in select situations including:
      - To evaluate women at risk for breast cancer who have mammographically dense breasts or breast implants or scars that limit the sensitivity of mammography[24]

- To detect unsuspected multifocal, multicentric, or bilateral breast cancer in women with newly diagnosed breast cancer[25]
- To detect the presence or absence of metastatic disease in the axillary lymph nodes
- To detect an occult breast primary in a patient with metastatic disease in the axillary nodes and normal mammography, sonography, and clinical breast exam[26]
- To distinguish benign from malignant mammographic lesions without biopsy[27]

c. Current Limitations

   i. Sensitivity depends on lesion size, with limited ability to detect small lesions[28]
- 97% for lesions > 1 cm
- 50% or less for lesions < 1 cm

   ii. Same sources of false-positives as mammography, including:
- Fibradenomata[24,25,27–30]
- Fibrocystic changes[24,28,29]
- Proliferative ductal epithelial hyperplasia [25]
- Breast abscess[29]

   iii. Lesion Localization
- If Tc-99m sestamibi scanning identifies a lesion that is not visible on traditional breast imaging modalities, there is currently no method to localize or mark this area for surgical excision.

d. Future Possibilities

   i. Tc-99m sestamibi scanning's ultimate role in breast imaging is still being defined. At our institution, we no longer perform Tc-99m sestamibi breast imaging because we did not feel that it offered clinically useful information beyond that offered by conventional breast imaging.

VII. Summary

A. Breast imaging is an essential component of screening for breast cancer and of evaluating women with breast symptoms. The conventional breast imaging methods of mammography and ultrasonography remain the foundation of breast imaging. Newer breast imaging techniques that continue to be evaluated include breast MRI, breast PET scanning, and scintimammography.

References

1. Fletcher SW. Why question screening mammography for women in their forties? In: Jackson VP, ed. Breast imaging. *Radiol Clin N Am* Philadelphia, PA: WB Saunders. 1995;33: 1259–1271.

2. Kopans DB. The positive predictive value of mammography. *Am J Roentgen AJR* 1992;158:521–526.

3. Jackson VP. Breast sonography. In: *Diagnosis of diseases of the breast.* Philadelphia, PA: WB Saunders; 1997:185–196.

4. Fornage BD, Coan JD, David CL. Ultrasound-guided needle biopsy of the breast and other interventional procedures. *Radiol Clin North Am* 1992;30:167–185. Philadelphia, PA: WB Saunders.

5. Parker SH, Lovin JD, Jobe WE, et al. Stereotactic breast biopsy with a biopsy gun. *Radiology* 1990;176:741–747.

6. Parker SH, Lovin JD, Jobe WE, et al. Nonpalpable breast lesions: stereotactic automated large-core biopsies. *Radiology* 1991;180:403–407.

7. Heywang-Kobrunner SH, Viehweg P, Heinig A, Kuchler CH. Contrast-enhanced MRI of the breast: accuracy, value, controversies, solutions. *Eur J Radiol* 1997;24:94–108.

8. Coons TA. MRI's role in assessing and managing breast disease. *Radio Tech* 1996;67:311–336.

9. Harms SE, Flamig DP, Hesley KL, et al. MR imaging of the breast with rotating delivery of excitation off resonance: clinical experience with pathologic correlation. *Radiology* 1993;187:493–501.

10. Nunes LW, Schnall MD, Orel SG, et al. Breast MR imaging: interpretation model. *Radiology* 1997;202:833–841.

11. Hulka CA, Edminster WB, Smith BL, et al. Dynamic echo-planar imaging of the breast: experience in diagnosing breast carcinoma and correlation with tumor angiogenesis. *Radiology* 1997;205:837–842.

12. Kaiser WA, Zeitler E. MR imaging of the breast: fast imaging sequences with and without Gd-DTPA. *Radiology* 1989;170:681–686.

13. Hulka CA, Smaith BL, Sgroi DC, et al. Benign and malignant breast lesions: differentiation with echo-planar MR imaging. *Radiology* 1995;197:33–38.

14. Servais F, Blocklet DC, Seret AE, et al. Differentiation between benign and malignant breast lesions with MR imaging and scintimammography. *Radiology* 1997;205:283–284.

15. Wahl RL, Cody R, Hutchins GD, et al. Primary and metastatic breast carcinoma: initial clinical evaluation with PET with the radiolabeled glucose analogue2-[18F]-fluoro-deoxy-2-D-glucose (FDG). *Radiology* 1991;179:765–770.

16. Adler LP, Crowe JP, Al-Kaisi NK, et al. Evaluation of breast masses and axillary lymph nodes with [18F]2-deoxy-2-fluoro-D-glucose PET. *Radiology* 1993;187:743–750.

17. Nieweg OE, Kim EE, Wong WH, et al. Positron emission tomography with fluorine-18-deoxy-glucose in the detection and staging of breast cancer. *Cancer* 1993;71:3920–3925.

18. Wahl RL, Helvie MA, Chang AE, et al. Detection of breast cancer in women after augmentation mammoplasty using fluorine-18-fluorodeoxyglucose-PET. *J Nucl Med* 1994;35:872–875.

19. Bassa P, Kim EE, Inoue T, et al. Evaluation of preoperative chemotherapy using PET with fluorine-18-fluorodeoxyglucose in breast cancer. *J Nucl Med* 1996;37:931–938.

20. Scheidhauer K, Scharl A, Pietrzyk U, et al. Qualitative [18F]FDG positron emission tomography in primary breast cancer: clinical relevance and practicability. *Eur J Nucl Med* 1996;23:618–623.

21. Bender H, Kirst J, Palmedo H, et al. Value of 18 fluoro-deoxyglucose positron emission tomography in staging of recurrent breast carcinoma. *Anticancer Res* 1997;177:1687–1692.

22. Adler DD, Wahl RL. New methods for imaging the breast: techniques, findings, and potential. *Am J Roentgen AJR* 1995;164:19–30.

23. Wahl RL. Nuclear medicine techniques in breast imaging. *Semin Ultrasound CT & MRI.* 1996;17:494–505.

24. Khalkhali I, Cutrone JA, Mena IG, et al. Scintimammography: the complementary role of Tc-99m sestamibi prone breast imaging for the diagnosis of breast carcinoma. *Radiology* 1995;196:421–426.

25. Fenlon HM, Phelan NC, O'Sullivan PO, et al. Benign versus malignant breast disease: comparison of contrast-enhanced MR imaging and Tc-99m tetrosfosmin scintimammography. *Radiology* 1997;205:214–220.

26. Mena FJ, Mena I, Diggles L, et al. Design and assessment of a scintigraphy-guided biplane localization technique for breast tumours: a phantom study. *Nucl Med Commun* 1996;17:717–723.

27. Carril JM, Gomez-Barquin R, Quirce R, et al. Contribution of Tc-99m MIBI scintimammography to the diagnosis of non-palpable breast lesions in relation to mammographic probability of malignancy. *Anticancer Res* 1997;17:1677–1682.

28. Scopinaro F, Ierardi M, Porfiri LM, et al. Tc-99m MIBI prone scintimammography in patients with high and intermediate risk mammography. *Anticancer Res* 1997;17:1635–1638.

29. Helbich TH, Becherer A, Trattnig S, et al. Differentiation of benign and malignant breast lesions: MR imaging versus Tc-99m sestamibi scintimammography. *Radiology* 1997;202:421–429.

30. Lam WW, Yang WT, Chan YL, et al. Role of MIBI breast scintigraphy in evaluation of palpable breast lesions. *Br J Radiol* 1996;69:1152–1158.

chapter 6

Ductal Lavage

Joyce A. O'Shaughnessy, MD
Codirector, Breast Cancer Research
Director, Breast Cancer Prevention Research
Baylor-Charles A. Sammons Cancer Center
Texas Oncology, PA, US Oncology
Dallas, TX

I.   **Ductal Lavage: The Procedure**

A. Ductal lavage is a procedure developed to enhance the ease and efficiency of collecting breast epithelial cells for cytologic analysis.[1]

B. Technique.

1. *Topical anesthetic cream, for example, EMLA cream (i.e., 2.5% lidocaine – 2.5% prilocaine, Astra USA, Westborough, MA) is applied to the nipple with an occlusive dressing for at least 1 hour.*

2. *The nipple is scrubbed with a dekeratinizing mild abrasive gel (Omni Prep Skin Prep; D.O. Weaver & Co., Aurora, CO).*

3. *After at least one minute of breast self-massage, nipple aspiration is performed by placing a suction cup attached to a syringe (Cytyc, Topsfield, MA) (Figure 6.1) over the nipple and applying 10 to 15 ml of suction (Figure 6.2). The lactiferous sinus is then manually compressed. Repeat steps until duct fluid is elicited or it is determined that the breast will not yield fluid.*

4. *High-risk women whose breasts do not yield fluid may be invited to return for repeated nipple aspiration.*

FIGURE 6.1   **Aspirator**

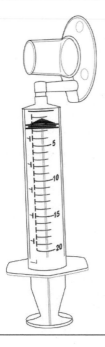

FIGURE 6.2	Aspiration

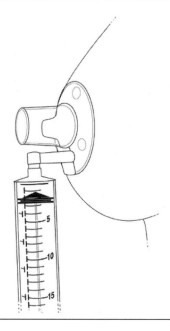

5. All fluid-yielding ducts should undergo ductal lavage to determine whether atypical breast epithelial cells are present.

6. A separate microcatheter (Cytyc, Topsfield, MA) is used to cannulate each duct to avoid cellular cross-contamination (see Figure 6.3).

7. The microcatheter (which may be lubricated with lidocaine jelly) is inserted 1 to 1.5 cm into the duct, past the duct sphincter, and 1 to 3 ml of 1% lidocaine without epinephrine is infused into the duct to provide anesthesia.

8. Approximately 3 to 6 ml of sterile normal saline is infused into the duct, and then the breast is compressed to facilitate recovery of ductal fluid into the collection chamber of the catheter. This sequence is repeated several times instilling about 10 to 15 cc of normal saline and collecting approximately 5 cc of effluent (see Figure 6.4).

9. The location of each lavaged duct is marked on a 64-square nipple grid to allow for future cannulation of the same duct.

10. The ductal lavage effluent is placed into tubes filled halfway with Cytolyt to preserve and fix the cells. Cytology specimens should be collected and analyzed separately for each duct.

FIGURE 6.3   Microcatheter

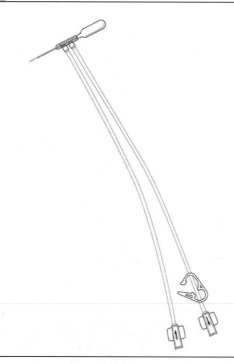

11. The ductal lavage fluid is processed using the Thin Prep technique (Cytyc, Topsfield, MA) for cytologic interpretation.

C. Cytologic Interpretation.

1. The diagnostic criteria and interpretations are very similar to those established by the 1997 National Cancer Institute Consensus Criteria for Breast Fine-Needle Aspiration Biopsy.[2]

2. The five diagnostic categories are:

a. Inadequate cellular material for diagnosis (ICMD, i.e., samples with fewer than 10 epithelial cells or unacceptable technical quality)

b. Benign

c. Mild atypia (representing atypical hyperplasia, usual hyperplasia, or proliferative papillary lesions or possibly low-grade DCIS)

d. Marked atypia (cells that have some but not all of the features of malignancy and may suggest high-grade atypical hyperplasia, ductal carcinoma in situ, or a florid papillomatosis pattern)

e. Malignant

| **FIGURE 6.4** | Lavage |

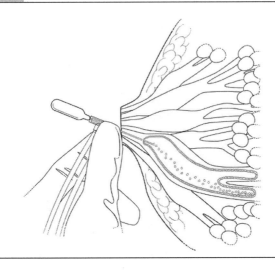

3. A web-based tutorial for cytology interpretation of the ductal lavage specimens has been established by the University of California, San Francisco (UCSF). Certification of pathologists involves their taking this tutorial and having their initial specimens interpreted as atypical double-read at UCSF, as well as any specimens called malignant.

4. It is important that ductal lavage specimens be interpreted by pathologists who have taken the web-based tutorial and who are participating in the quality control process ongoing at UCSF.

D. Rationale for Performing Ductal Lavage.

1. Both ductal and lobular invasive breast cancer arise from the ductal and lobular epithelial cells that line the complex, branching breast ductal system.

2. Breast carcinogenesis has a long subclinical period of intraepithelial neoplasia (IEN) characterized by progression of cytologically normal-appearing cells that have accumulated molecular abnormalities to usual hyperplasia, atypical hyperplasia to ductal and lobular carcinoma in situ.

3. Except for ductal carcinoma in situ (DCIS), breast IEN is not generally detectable on physical examination or on mammography.

4. The presence of biopsy-proven atypical hyperplasia[3] or cytologically atypical cells detected by NAF[4] or breast fine-

needle aspiration (FNA) increases the risk for developing breast cancer approximately fivefold. This risk increases to elevenfold to eighteenfold if the woman also has a family history of breast cancer[3,4,5]

5. Ductal lavage has been developed as a minimally invasive way to facilitate retrieval of intraductal epithelial cells to identify women who are at markedly elevated risk of developing breast cancer because of the presence of atypical epithelial cells.

6. The primary purpose of ductal lavage is risk stratification, that is, to provide additional information to women who are at elevated risk on the basis of their 5-year Gail risk score, and to further stratify risk into those women who are at elevated versus high risk.

7. Five years of tamoxifen treatment, 20 mg QD, has been shown to reduce breast cancer risk by 86% in women with biopsy-proven atypical hyperplasia,[6] which is generally an estrogen and progesterone receptor-positive lesion.[7]

8. Women who are found to have atypical epithelial cells on ductal lavage are excellent candidates for tamoxifen risk reduction therapy because the benefits generally greatly outweigh the risks.

E. Pivotal Ductal Lavage versus Nipple Aspiration Fluid (NAF) Study[1]

1. Dooley, et al. published their results in 507 women at elevated risk for breast cancer on the basis of a 5-year Gail risk score of 1.7% or greater, previous history of breast cancer, or known BRCA1/2 mutation carrier who underwent both nipple aspiration and ductal lavage.

2. Cytologic analysis was performed on NAF specimens from 417 subjects (83% of the high-risk women had at least one fluid-yielding duct on nipple aspiration) and from 383 subjects who had fluid-yielding ducts that could be successfully cannulated for ductal lavage.

3. Both NAF and ductal lavage were safe and well tolerated. On a 100-mm pain scale with 0 representing no pain and 100 representing extreme pain, the women rated ductal lavage as having an average pain score of 22.

4. Seventy-three percent of the NAF specimens were ICMD (contained fewer than 10 epithelial cells) while only 22% of the ductal lavage specimens were ICMD.

5. NAF specimens contained an average of 120 cells obtained per breast while the ductal lavage fluid contained an average of 13,500 cells per duct. Cytology interpretation is facilitated by more cellular preparations.

6. Twenty-four percent of the high-risk women had abnormal cells detected in their ductal lavage specimens (atypical or malignant) compared to 10% of the NAF specimens (Table 6.1). Ductal lavage was 3.2 times more sensitive in detecting abnormal cells than was NAF when samples from the same breast were compared.

TABLE 6.1	Distribution of Cytologic Diagnoses Among High-Risk Women Having Both Ductal Lavage and Nipple Aspiration	
Cytologic Diagnosis	Ductal Lavage	NAF
ICMD	84 (22%)	306 (73%)
Benign	207 (54%)	70 (17%)
Mild atypia	66 (17%)	27 (6%)
Marked atypia	24 (6%)	12 (3%)
Malignant	2 (<1%)	2 (<1%)
Total	383 subjects	417 subjects

*ICMD—insufficient cellular material for diagnosis (fewer than 10 epithelial cells)

Dooley WC, Ljung BM, Veronesi U, et al. Ductal lavage for detection of cellular atypia in women at high risk for breast cancer. *J Natl Cancer Inst* 2001;93:1624–1632.

7. Interestingly, the 24% incidence of atypical cells found in the ductal lavage specimens in the high-risk women is approximately the same as the 21% incidence of cytologic atypia found by Fabian, et al. in high-risk women who underwent bilateral breast periareolar, random FNA.

8. This suggests that lavaging the fluid-yielding ducts only (and not the nonfluid-yielding ducts) leads to detection of atypical cells in an expected proportion of high-risk subjects and that the fluid-yielding ducts are more likely to contain breast IEN than are nonfluid-yielding ducts.

F. Candidates for Ductal Lavage.

1. A woman should be offered ductal lavage only if she is at elevated risk for breast cancer and if a finding of atypical cells on cytology would change her clinical management.

2. Changes in clinical management of the high-risk woman that could occur based on a finding of cellular atypical include:

   a. Taking tamoxifen risk reduction therapy for five years
   b. Participation in the NSABP STAR (Study of Tamoxifen and Raloxifene) or other clinical trial
   c. Stopping hormone replacement therapy (HRT)
   d. Increased breast surveillance with physical exams and breast imaging studies
   e. Prophylactic mastectomy for women with a known BRCA1 or BRCA2 germline mutation

3. Women who are appropriate candidates for ductal lavage include those who are at elevated risk for breast cancer based on:

   a. A 5-year Gail risk score ≥ 1.7%
   b. Two or more second-degree affected relatives with breast cancer[8] (Offering ductal lavage to these potential candidates is not yet supported by evidence-based consensus at present.)
   c. Having taken combined estrogen and progesterone hormone replacement therapy for greater than 10 years[9]

   d. Remote history of biopsy-proven atypical ductal or lobular hyperplasia (ADH/ALH), lobular carcinoma in situ (LCIS),[7] and unwilling to take standard tamoxifen therapy without information that atypical cells remain in a breast duct

   e. Known BRCA1/2 mutation or suspected BRCA1/2 mutation (strong family history with two or more first-degree relatives with breast and/or ovarian cancer) if a finding of atypical cells would influence clinical management, for example, instituting tamoxifen therapy or prophylactic mastectomy

4. *The purpose of ductal lavage is to stratify appropriate candidates into those at substantially elevated risk (based on the presence of atypical breast epithelial cells) and those with only benign cytology who retain only their original elevated risk. For example, a finding of atypical breast cells in a woman not previously known to have atypical hyperplasia or LCIS approximately doubles her 5-year and lifetime Gail risk of developing breast cancer.*

5. *While most women who are at elevated or high risk for breast cancer based on the preceding risk factors are good candidates for risk reduction interventions, many decline to stop their HRT or to take tamoxifen because of side effects.[10] A finding of atypical cells on ductal lavage significantly further increases a woman's risk, thereby increasing the benefit to risk ratio for tamoxifen therapy.*

6. *Women who are not appropriate candidates for ductal lavage include:*

   a. Those with an abnormal breast examination, mammogram, or other breast imaging study. Such a finding requires standard evaluation and biopsy. Ductal lavage is *not* a diagnostic tool to detect cancer.

   b. High-risk women with dense breasts on mammogram who either wish or require another breast screening evaluation. Ductal lavage is *not* a screening test for occult breast cancer.

   c. High-risk women with a history of ER/PR-positive breast cancer or DCIS, biopsy-proven ADH, ALH, or LCIS who are willing to take standard tamoxifen risk reduction therapy. A finding of atypical cells on ductal lavage *does not* further elevate such a woman's already high risk. Such patients should be treated with tamoxifen for five years provided the patient does not have a medical condition contraindicating tamoxifen therapy.

   d. Women at elevated breast cancer risk who have a history of a deep vein thrombosis, pulmonary embolus, history of invasive endometrial cancer, recent transient ischemic attack, cerebrovascular accident, active angina, or recent myocardial infarction are *not* candidates for tamoxifen therapy. A finding of atypical cells will probably not lead to the use of tamoxifen for risk reduction. These women should not undergo ductal lavage unless a finding of atypical breast cells would change their breast surveillance program or, in a woman with a known BRCA1/2 mutation, would lead to prophylactic mastectomy.

   e. Women taking tamoxifen for a history of invasive breast cancer, DCIS, ADH, ALH, LCIS, a family history of breast cancer, or an elevated 5-year Gail risk score.

   f. There is no proven role for ductal lavage in serially monitoring breast cytology in high-risk women who are taking tamoxifen or who have taken five years of tamoxifen.

| FIGURE 6.5 | Ductal Lavage Algorithm |

Benign ➡	Repeat ductal lavage in 1–3 years
Mildly Atypical ➡	Strongly consider tamoxifen or prevention trial unless contraindicated
	Repeat ductal lavage in 6–12 months to confirm findings
Markedly Atypical ➡	Repeat ductal lavage to confirm findings
	Additional imaging (ductogram, MRI, ductoscopy)
	Biopsy if abnormality found
	Strongly consider tamoxifen or prevention trial unless contraindicated
Malignant ➡	Repeat ductal lavage to confirm findings
	Additional imaging (ductogram, MRI, ductoscopy)
	Surgical excision if an abnormality is found
	Strongly consider tamoxifen or prevention unless contraindicated
ICMD ➡	Repeat lavage at next opportunity; if again ICMD and good fluid exchange observed, follow up in 1–3 years

g. There is no proven therapy for breast atypical hyperplasia in patients who have already been treated with tamoxifen.

h. It is not known whether tamoxifen therapy changes the cytologic findings of atypia on ductal lavage and, if so, over what period of time.

II. Ductal Lavage Findings: Clinical Implications

A. Figure 6.5 summarizes a clinical management pathway based on the cytology results on ductal lavage. This pathway represents the consensus opinion of 17 physicians who are experienced in breast cancer risk assessment and ductal lavage.[11]

B. Inadequate Cellular Material for Diagnosis (ICMD).

1. This is defined as having fewer than 10 breast epithelial cells in the ductal lavage fluid for cytologic diagnosis.

2. This finding is generally due to a technical problem with lavage such as duct perforation or failure to seat the lavage catheter beyond the duct sphincter.

3. However, a finding of ICMD may also result from lavage of an atrophic or normal breast duct. For a first diagnosis of ICMD from a fluid-yielding duct, ductal lavage should be repeated.

4. For a second diagnosis of ICMD in the same duct, especially with good fluid exchange in the catheter during lavage, this duct may be followed the same way as a finding of benign cells.

C. Benign Cells.

1. A finding of only benign cells on ductal lavage has not yet been proven to lower a high-risk woman's risk of developing breast cancer.

2. Such a woman, therefore, still retains her elevated risk status, and antiestrogen therapy should be considered. It is not

known what the optimal interval for serial lavage is in a high-risk woman with benign cytology to monitor her for the development of atypical cells.

3. However, it is reasonable to consider repeating the lavage in one to three years if the high-risk woman has not begun antiestrogen risk reduction therapy.

D. Atypical Cells.

1. Tamoxifen therapy for five years is recommended for women with atypical cytology on breast lavage or participation in a breast cancer prevention clinical trial.

2. Women on HRT should be counseled about the risks and benefits of HRT given the finding of atypia.

3. It is reasonable to recommend that a woman stop HRT and take tamoxifen, as the combination has not been definitively shown to be effective in reducing risk.

4. A finding of atypical cells on lavage is not an indication for surgical excision unless an abnormality is noted on physical exam or mammogram.

E. Markedly Atypical Cells.

1. Markedly atypical cells have several, but not all, of the features of malignancy.

2. If a high-risk woman is found to have markedly atypical cells on lavage, lavage of the same duct should be repeated to confirm the finding.

3. While this cytologic finding may be indicative of an occult invasive cancer or DCIS, the markedly atypical cells may also represent benign disease such as ADH or papillomatosis with or without atypia.

4. Ductography is recommended to determine whether an intraluminal filling defect is present which can be localized for surgical excision.

5. If ductoscopy is available, this procedure may be useful in localizing the intraductal pathology for excision.

6. Additional imaging studies such as breast magnetic resonance imaging, ultrasound, or digital mammography may be warranted to search for a suspicious lesion. Any suspicious lesion should be biopsied.

7. In the absence of finding a suspicious lesion to biopsy, tamoxifen therapy is recommended for women with markedly atypical cells.

8. Surgical exploration of the ductal system is not recommended as, in the absence of a filling defect on ductography or ductoscopy, it may be impossible to identify the abnormal lesion due to the widely branching nature of the ductal system.

9. There is not at present a well-established relationship between a finding of markedly atypical cells on lavage and a pathologic diagnosis of malignancy.

F. Malignant Cells.

1. A finding of malignant cells on ductal lavage is expected to occur in <0.5% of high-risk women. In this case, lavage of the same duct should be repeated to confirm the finding.

2. As described previously for a finding of markedly atypical cells, ductography and ductoscopy, if available are recommended to identify a potentially suspicious lesion for biopsy.

3. Additional breast imaging studies are also indicated to determine whether a suspicious lesion that is amenable to biopsy can be identified.

4. If no suspicious lesion is found, surgical duct exploration or mastectomy is not recommended because it may be impossible to localize a small lesion in the widely branching ductal system and because a correlation between malignant cytology on lavage and malignant histology on biopsy has not been established.

5. Tamoxifen risk reduction therapy is recommended as is careful breast imaging and examination surveillance.

III. **Incorporating Ductal Lavage into the Management of the High-Risk Woman**

A. Figures 6.6 through 6.8 summarize the current thinking of breast cancer risk assessment experts who have incorporated ductal lavage into their clinical management of high-risk women.

B. Figures 6.6 through 6.8 describe the risk factors that place women into the categories of very high risk (relative risk fivefold or greater), elevated or high risk (twofold to fourfold elevated relative risk), and average risk (less than twofold relative risk).

FIGURE 6.6 **Risk Management Strategy**

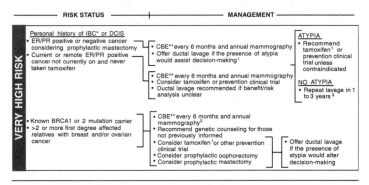

*IBC = Invasive Breast Cancer **CBE = Clinical Breast Exam

[1] Sufficient evidence is not available at this time to make a definitive recommendation.

[2] Consider increased imaging surveillance such as breast MRI or ultrasound and initiation of mammography before age 40.

[3] These patients should also be considered for prevention clinical trials.

*Risk Assessment Working Group: Terry Bevers, Laura Esserman, Linda Frame, Darius Francescatti, Anne-Renee Hartman, Alan Hollingsworth, Suzanne Klimberg, Monica Morrow, Wendy Mikkelson, David Nathanson, Lisa Newman, Joyce O'Shaughnessy, Freya Schnabel, Eva Singletary, and Victor Vogel, Chair.

C. Figures 6.6 through 6.8 also summarize clinical pathways that can assist clinicians in evaluating and managing the high-risk woman.

D. Ductal lavage can be utilized in several of these pathways if the benefit/risk analysis of tamoxifen, participation in a breast cancer prevention clinical trial, or prophylactic mastectomy for known or suspected BRCA1/2 mutation carriers is not clear.

E. Ductal lavage is indicated only if a finding of atypical breast epithelial cells would facilitate clinical decision-making and would likely change clinical management.

F. These clinical pathways represent the consensus opinion of breast cancer risk assessment physicians. Where sufficient evidence does not exist to make a definitive recommendation, this is indicated as a footnote.

IV. **Ongoing Evaluation of Ductal Lavage**

A. Ductal lavage practitioners are participating in the Ductal Lavage Outcomes Tracking System (DLOTS), which is prospectively evaluating the clinical outcomes of high-risk women who undergo ductal lavage.

B. Outcomes being tracked are changes in clinical management that result from lavage including beginning antiestrogen therapy, stopping HRT, enhancing breast imaging surveillance, undergoing a breast biopsy, or a pathologic finding of atypical hyperplasia, LCIS, DCIS, or invasive cancer.

FIGURE 6.7   **Risk Management Strategy**

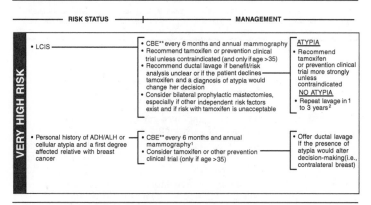

*IBC = Invasive Breast Cancer **CBE = Clinical Breast Exam*

[1] *Consider increased imaging surveillance such as breast MRI or ultrasound and initiation of mammography before age 40.*

[2] *These patients should also be considered for prevention clinical trials.*

Risk Assessment Working Group: Terry Bevers, Laura Esserman, Linda Frame, Darius Francescatti, Anne-Renee Hartmann, Alan Hollingsworth, Suzanne Klimberg, Monica Morrow, Wendy Mikkelson, David Nathanson, Lisa Newman, Joyce O'Shaughnessy, Freya Schnabel, Eva Singletary, and Victor Vogel, Chair.

FIGURE 6.8   Risk Management Strategy

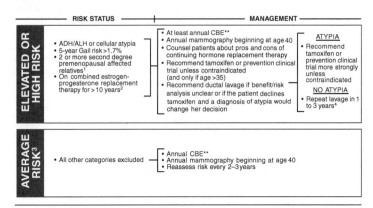

*IBC = Invasive Breast Cancer **CBE = Clinical Breast Exam

[1] For more accurate risk assessment of mixtures of 1st and 2nd degree relatives consult the Claus model.

[2] For more accurate risk assessment of scenarios of first and second degree affected relatives, consult the Claus model.

[3] More than half of women diagnosed with breast cancer have no known risk factors.

[4] These patients should also be considered for prevention clinical trials.

*Risk Assessment Working Group: Terry Bevers, Laura Esserman, Linda Frame, Darius Francescatti, Anne-Renee Hartmann, Alan Hollingsworth, Suzanne Klimberg, Monica Morrow, Wendy Mikkelson, David Nathanson, Lisa Newman, Joyce O'Shaughnessy, Freya Schnabel, Eva Singletary, and Victor Vogel, Chair.

C. The web-based DLOTS is available to all ductal lavage practitioners and allows for easy entry of patient demographic information, ductal lavage findings, and clinical management/outcomes.

 1. DLOTS must be IRB-approved at each institution and informed consent of participants is required.

 2. Ductal lavage practitioners are able to track their own ductal lavage results over time, as well as access the national lavage database using DLOTS.

 3. This important prospective national outcomes study will provide valuable information about the clinical utility of ductal lavage in high-risk women. The DLOTS web site is http://www.outcomessciences.com.

D. Ductal lavage is also being utilized as a research tool to investigate the molecular characteristics of the breast epithelial cells and proteins in the lavage effluent. Promising molecular biomarkers such as loss of heterozygosity of chromosomes,[12] methylated genes,[13] and abnormal protein components by mass spectroscopy[14] are being evaluated with the aims of diagnosing occult breast cancer early and of differentiating atypical cells that have a high risk of progressing to invasive cancer from those with a lower risk.

E. Clinical trials are also underway to serially monitor atypical breast epithelial cells in high-risk women who are taking an antiestrogen or a novel investigational risk reduction agent such as celecoxib. It is important to study the effects of these interventions on the patterns of cellular atypia to determine whether there is a correlation between the development of clinical breast cancer and apoptosis or persistence of atypical breast cells.

References

1. Dooley WC, Ljung BM, Veronesi U, et al. Ductal lavage for detection of cellular atypia in women at high risk for breast cancer. *J Natl Cancer Inst* 2001;93:1624–1632.

2. The uniform approach to breast fine-needle aspirate biopsy. NIH Consensus Development Conference. *Am J Surg* 1997;174:371–385.

3. Dupont WD, Parl FF, Hartmann WH, Brinton LA, Winfield AC, Worrell JA. Breast cancer risk associated with proliferative breast disease and atypical hyperplasia. *Cancer* 1993;71A:1258–1265.

4. Wrensch MR, Petrakis NL, Miike R, et al. Breast cancer risk in women with abnormal cytology in nipple aspirates of breast fluid. *J Natl Cancer Inst* 2001;93:1791–1798.

5. Fabian CJ, Kimler BF, Zalles CM, Klemp JR, Kamel S, Zeiger S. Short-term breast cancer prediction by random periareolar fine-needle aspiration cytology and the Gail risk model. *J Natl Cancer Inst* 2000;92:1217–1227.

6. Fisher B, Costantino JP, Wickerham DL, Redmond CK, Kavanah M, Cronin WM. Tamoxifen for prevention of breast cancer: report of the National Surgical Adjuvant Breast and Bowel Project P-1 Study. *J Natl Cancer Inst* 1998;90:1371–1388.

7. Khan SA, Rogers MA, Obando JA, Tamsen A. Estrogen receptor expression of benign breast epithelium and its association with breast cancer. *Cancer Res* 1994;54:993–997.

8. Claus EB, Schildkraut JM, Thompson WD, Risch NJ. The genetic attributable risk of breast and ovarian cancer. *Cancer* 1996;77:2318–2224.

9. Writing Group for the Women's Health Initiative Investigators. Risks and benefits of estrogen plus progestin in healthy postmenopausal women—principal results from the Women's Health Initiative randomized controlled trial. *JAMA* 2002;288:321–333.

10. Port ER, Montgomery LL, Heerdt AS, Borgen PI. Patient reluctance toward tamoxifen use for breast cancer primary prevention. *Ann Surg Oncol* 2001;8:580–584.

11. O'Shaughnessy JA, Ljung BM, Dooley WC, et al. Ductal lavage and the clinical management of women at high risk for breast carcinoma. A Commentary. *Cancer* 2002;94:292–298.

12. Gherardi G, Marveggio C. Cytologic score and DNA-image analysis in the classification of borderline breast lesions: a prospective study on 47 fine-needle aspirates. *Diagn Cytopath* 1999;20:212–218.

13. Evron E, Dooley WC, Umbricht CB, et al. Detection of breast cancer cells in ductal lavage fluid by methylation-specific PCR. *Lancet* 2001;357:1335–1336.

14. Paweletz CP, Li F, Trock BJ, Petricoin EF, Liotta LA. Diagnosis of breast cancer from nipple aspirate fluids based on multiparametric proteomic analysis [abstract 683]. *Proc Amer Assoc Cancer Res* 2002;43:136.

chapter 7

Chemoprevention

Jeanne Lebish, CRNP
Kristen Kotsko, RN, BSN
University of Pittsburgh Cancer Institute/
Magee-Womens Hospital
Pittsburgh, PA

I.   **Introduction to Chemoprevention**
  A. Definition: "the use of specific natural or synthetic chemical agents to reverse, suppress, or prevent the progression of premalignant lesions to invasive carcinoma."[1]
  B. Carcinogenesis is defined as the transformation of a normal cell into a malignant cell.
  C. In July 1998, NCI's Division of Cancer Prevention (DCP) created the Chemoprevention Implementation Group (CIG) to further define and guide research in the field of chemoprevention.[2]
  D. High-risk women can be defined by the Gail model.[3]
     1. *An accurate method of quantifying a woman's risk of developing breast cancer with a risk of breast cancer at least 1.7% in five years is considered high risk.*
     2. *Risk factors are entered into a computer program or hand-held device and given a value that is used to compute 5-year and lifetime risks of breast cancer.*
        a. As a woman ages, risk increases.
        b. Age at menarche younger than 12 years.
        c. Age at first live birth 30 years and older.
        d. Number of first-degree relatives with breast cancer, that is, mother, sister, daughter (does not take into account male breast cancer or other relatives). There are other models that calculate breast cancer risk by taking these relatives into consideration.
        e. Number of breast biopsies—as the number increases, the likelihood that an abnormality will exist increases.
           i. A woman with a biopsy diagnosis of lobular carcinoma *in situ* (LCIS) experienced an annual risk for invasive breast cancer of 1.3% per year in the Breast Cancer Prevention Trial.[4]
           ii. A biopsy diagnosis of atypical ductal hyperplasia increases a woman's risk two-fold.

II. **Role of Hormones in Chemoprevention**
  A. Estrogen production in the ovaries declines with age and finally ceases causing menopause (decrease of estradiol with increasing FSH and LH).
  B. With declining estrogen levels in the body, women begin to suffer from vasomotor hot flashes, night sweats, and bone loss.
  C. Estrogen is known to fuel the growth of certain types of breast and endometrial cancers.
  D. Estrogen has not been found to prevent the progression of coronary atherosclerosis as previously thought.
  E. Estrogen production continues in postmenopausal women from the adrenal glands with conversion in adipose tissue to a weaker estrogen called estrone.
  F. Estrogen target tissues.
     1. *Hypothalmo-pituitary axis controls menses via a feedback mechanism*
     2. *Maintains bone density*
     3. *Causes proliferation of breast tissue*

4. *Uterus*

    a. Estrogen regulates the uterine tissue by preparing it for progesterone stimulation following ovulation with anticipation of implantation of a fertilized ovum; without implantation, menstruation occurs.

    b. Following menopause, the uterine lining may proliferate with unopposed estrogen stimulation.

5. *Vaginal and urogenital mucosa*

6. *Liver (cholesterol and lipids)*

III. Selective Estrogen Receptor Modulators (SERMs)

A. Tamoxifen (Nolvadex®)

1. *It is a triphenylethylene that has been shown to be species-specific, tissue-specific, and disease-specific.*

2. *Mechanism of action.*

    a. Binds estrogen receptors.

    b. In postmenopausal women, treatment with tamoxifen results in the upregulation of the proportion of ductal cells expressing estrogen receptor.

    c. Pharmacology.

        i. Half-life of 9 to 12 hours after initial dose

        ii. Half-life rises to 7 days after chronic use

    d. Dosage.

        i. 10 mg, twice daily, orally or 20 mg, once daily, orally.

        ii. Chemoprevention is recommended for five years utilizing tamoxifen as the only currently approved drug for the reduction of breast cancer risk.

3. *In the adjuvant setting.*

    a. First line treatment.

    b. Tamoxifen has been the standard of care with years of data available.

    c. Dosage: 10 mg, twice daily, orally or 20 mg daily, orally.

    d. Used for both premenopausal and postmenopausal women.

    e. Treatment of choice with history of osteopenia or osteoporosis.

4. *Prevention setting use: Only approved agent by the U.S. Food and Drug Administration to reduce the incidence of breast cancer in high-risk women.*

B. Raloxifene HCL (Evista®)—a benzothiophene derivative that binds to the estrogen receptor

1. *MORE trial (Multiple Outcomes Raloxifene Evaluation).*[5]

    a. MORE was a randomized, placebo-controlled, double-blind trial that concluded in 1999, designed to determine whether raloxifene reduces the risk of fractures in postmenopausal women with osteoporosis.

    b. 7,705 women with a mean age of 66.5 years (the youngest being 31 years, and the oldest being 80 years) were randomized to the trial.

        i. Breast cancer risk factors were not routinely ascertained at baseline.

        ii. Eligible women for the MORE trial who had a low bone mineral density also have a notably lower increased risk for developing breast cancer.

    c. 95.7% of women randomized were Caucasian.

   d. The subjects received either 60 mg raloxifene, 120 mg
       raloxifene, or placebo.
       i.   2,557 women received raloxifene 60mg/day.
       ii. 2,572 women received raloxifene 120 mg/day.
   e. The primary endpoint was the development of osteoporosis.
   f. Breast density did not increase in women taking raloxifene
       following two years of therapy which is significant in that
       Raloxifene does not impede mammographic detection of
       new breast cancers.
   g. The secondary endpoint was the development of breast
       cancer.
       i.   After four years, 22 cases of breast cancer were
            confirmed among the 5,129 women who took raloxifene
            versus 39 cases among the 2,576 women who took the
            placebo.
       ii. 31 ER-positive invasive breast cancers were reported in
            the placebo group versus 10 ER-positive invasive breast
            cancers in the raloxifene groups.
   h. Women randomized to receive raloxifene in the MORE trial
       had a threefold increased incidence of thrombosis equal to
       the risk seen in the BCPT.
   i. Raloxifene reduced the risk of newly diagnosed invasive
       breast cancer by 72% and ER-positive invasive breast cancer
       by 84%.
   j. There was no significant difference between raloxifene 60 mg
       daily and 120 mg daily in either outcomes or side effects.
   k. Raloxifene blocked the estrogen receptor positive in estrogen
       receptor-positive breast cancer but showed no effect on
       estrogen receptor-negative breast cancers.
   l. It is speculated that women with detectable levels of
       estradiol may benefit more from raloxifene's reduction in
       breast cancer risk than women with undetectable estradiol
       levels.[6]

2. *Indicated for postmenopausal women to prevent and treat
    osteoporosis.*

3. *Increases bone density and reduces fractures in
    postmenopausal women.*

4. *Not FDA approved for chemoprevention of breast cancer.*

5. *Currently in clinical trial: STAR Trial (Study of Tamoxifen and
    Raloxifene) to evaluate reduction of breast cancer risk, along
    with its effect on osteoporosis and heart disease (see the
    following).*

6. *Dosage: 60 mg, once daily, orally.*

7. *Benefits versus risks.*
    a. Antiestrogenic effects seen in breast in limited data as
        secondary endpoint in postmenopausal women
    b. Increased risk of thromboembolic disease[7]

8. *Estrogenic effects.*
    a. Increases bone density in postmenopausal women
    b. Reduces total cholesterol by reducing LDL without effect on
        HDL—no reduction in coronary heart disease[8]

9. *Side effects.*
    a. Less likely to cause endometrial stimulation and/or result in
        endometrial cancer[7]
    b. Leg cramps

10. *Management of side effects (leg cramps).*
    a. Tonic water contains quinine and may provide relief.
    b. Calcium-magnesium supplements are available over the counter.

11. *Raloxifene Use for the Heart (RUTH) study.*
    a. Designed to evaluate the ability of raloxifene in preventing heart attacks, other cardiac events, and invasive breast cancers in postmenopausal women who are at risk for heart attack or coronary artery disease
    b. Enrolled 10,000 older women at risk for heart disease
    c. Results expected in 2004

12. *The Continuing Outcomes Relevant to Evista (CORE) trial is evaluating the long-term effects of raloxifene on reducing the incidence of breast cancer in postmenopausal women in the MORE trial.*

IV. **Clinical Trials Evaluating Chemoprevention for the Reduction of Breast Cancer Risk**

A. Breast Cancer Prevention Trial (BCPT)

1. *The National Cancer Institute, in collaboration with the National Surgical Adjuvant Breast and Bowel Project launched the Breast Cancer Prevention Trial (BCPT) in 1992 to evaluate the ability of tamoxifen to prevent breast cancer in women who were at increased risk.*[4]

2. *Women eligible for the trial were either older than 60 years at entry, were age 35 or older with a breast biopsy showing lobular carcinoma in situ, or were between the ages of 35 and 59 years with an estimated annual risk for developing breast cancer equal to that of a 60-year-old woman.*

3. *Risk was estimated using the Gail model developed by Gail and his colleagues.*

4. *13,388 premenopausal and postmenopausal women with an increased risk for breast cancer were randomly assigned to take either tamoxifen 20 mg per day or a placebo daily for five years.*

5. *Participants were unblinded early due to a statistical difference in the number of invasive breast cancers developed between the women on tamoxifen and the women on placebo.*

6. *Reduction in incidence of invasive breast cancer.*
    a. Through July 1998, a total of 368 invasive and noninvasive breast cancers occurred among 13,175 women with evaluable endpoints in BCPT.
    b. There were a total of 175 cases of invasive breast cancer in the placebo group as compared with 89 in the tamoxifen group (risk ratio 0.51, 95% confidence interval (CI) 0.39–0.66, $p < 0.00001$).
    c. The annual event rate for invasive breast cancer among women taking tamoxifen was 3.4 per 1,000 women compared with 6.8 per 1,000 women taking placebo.
    d. Reduced risk of developing invasive breast cancer occurred among all age groups in the trial. Risk ratios were:
        i. 0.56 for women ≤ 49 years of age;
        ii. 0.49 for women 50 to 59 years; and
        iii. 0.45 for women 60 years old or older.

e. A benefit was seen for women with a history of lobular carcinoma *in situ* (risk ratio 0.44, 95% CI 0.16–1.06).

f. For women with a history of atypical lobular or ductal hyperplasia, the risk ratio was markedly diminished at 0.14 (95% CI 0.03–0.47).

g. Reduced risk ratios were seen at all projected levels of risk and among women with one, two, or three or more first-degree relatives with a history of invasive breast cancer.

h. The reduction in the risk of invasive breast cancer was seen within the first year of the trial, and lower incidence rates for women taking tamoxifen compared with those taking placebo were seen for each subsequent year of the trial throughout six years of maximum follow-up at the time the results were reported.

i. The incidence rate of estrogen receptor-positive breast cancers was 5 per 1,000 women in the placebo group compared with only 1.6 per 1,000 women in the tamoxifen group, a 69% reduction.

j. Rates of estrogen receptor-negative tumors were not significantly different in the two treatment groups (1.46 per 1,000 women in the tamoxifen group compared with 1.20 per 1,000 women in the placebo group).

7. *No significant reduction in the rates of myocardial infarction, coronary artery bypass, ischemic heart disease, or angioplasty was noted in the BCPT.*

8. *Fracture rates.*

a. In BCPT, 955 women experienced bone fractures.

b. The incidence of osteoporotic fracture events involving the hip, spine, or lower radius was reduced 19% among women receiving tamoxifen.

c. Fewer osteoporotic events (combined hip, spine, and lower radius) occurred in women receiving tamoxifen than in those receiving placebo.

d. There was a 45% reduction in fractures of the hip.

e. Overall, 111 women in the tamoxifen arm experienced fractures at one or more sites as compared with 137 women in the placebo arm.

f. This represents a 19% reduction in the incidence of fractures when tamoxifen is compared with placebo.

9. *Incidence of invasive endometrial cancer.*

a. Increased incidence in the number of endometrial cancers noted in the women randomized to the tamoxifen arm of the trial.

b. Increase occurred more often in women age 50 and older.

c. All the endometrial cancers found were Stage I (localized disease) with none resulting in death.

d. Women who received tamoxifen in BCPT had a 2.5 times greater risk of developing invasive endometrial cancer than did women who received placebo.

e. The average annual rate was 2.3 per 1,000 women in the tamoxifen group and 0.9 per 1,000 women in the placebo group.

10. *Other Unfavorable Events.*[9]

a. There was an increase in the number of thromboembolic vascular events among women taking tamoxifen in the BCPT.

    b. There was a marginal increase of approximately 14% in the rate of cataract development among women who were free of cataracts at the time of entry into the BCPT. Event rates for cataract surgery were also increased for women taking tamoxifen when compared to those taking the placebo.

    c. Bothersome hot flashes were reported by 46% of women in the tamoxifen group compared with only 29% in the placebo group.

    d. Vaginal discharge reported as moderately bothersome or worse was seen in 29% of the tamoxifen group as compared with 13% of the placebo group.

    e. No other significant increase was noted in any other type of cancer, that is, colon, liver, or ovarian, among the women randomized to receive tamoxifen.

    f. The rates of thromboembolic events were increased threefold in women 50 and older in the women taking tamoxifen.

B. Royal Marsden Hospital Chemoprevention Trial[10]

  1. Trial opened for enrollment in 1986.

  2. Trial enrolled 2,494 women, 30 to 70 years of age, with a family history of breast cancer, women without a personal history of any cancer and/or thromboembolic venous event. Estrogen replacement therapy use was allowed during the trial.

  3. Twenty-six percent of women used estrogen replacement therapy with tamoxifen.

  4. Women were treated for an average of 70 months receiving either 20 mg of tamoxifen or placebo.

  5. Trial was unable to show any protective effect in healthy women following an 8-year follow-up and did not show any difference in the number of thromboembolic events between the two groups.

  6. Thirty-four patients in the tamoxifen arm of the trial developed breast cancer compared with 36 in the placebo arm.

  7. Of note: women who started HRT (hormone replacement therapy) during the trial had a reduced risk of breast cancer while women who were on HRT at the beginning of the trial had an increased risk.

  8. More women experienced adverse events in the tamoxifen group including hot flashes, gynecologic problems, menstrual irregularities, and mood changes.

  9. Four women in the tamoxifen group developed endometrial cancer compared with one from the placebo group.

  10. More patients discontinued therapy in the tamoxifen group than did the placebo group.

  11. This trial suggested that tamoxifen is not effective in lowering risk in women with low to moderate risk for developing breast cancer.

C. Italian Tamoxifen Prevention Study[11]

  1. Study began enrolling women in 1992 and randomized 5,408 women aged 35 to 70.

  2. Women were eligible only if they had a history of hysterectomy.

3. *Breast cancer risk was not evaluated for eligibility.*
4. *Women with a history of endometriosis or venous thromboembolic disease were excluded.*
5. *Estrogen replacement therapy was allowed.*
6. *Women were treated an average of 46 months.*
7. *Women were randomized to either tamoxifen 20 mg daily or placebo.*
8. *Trial closed prematurely due to a high rate of attrition.*
9. *Twenty-six percent of women dropped out with half dropping out within the first year.*
10. *No significant difference between the rates of breast cancer were noted for the two groups.*
11. *There were 22 cases of breast cancer in the placebo group with 19 cases in the tamoxifen group.*
12. *Venous thromboembolism, superficial phlebitis, and hypertriglyceridemia occurred more frequently in the women treated with tamoxifen.*
13. *There were nine deaths in the placebo group and six deaths in the tamoxifen group.*
14. *Trial demonstrated that tamoxifen is not effective in lowering risk in women with low to moderate risk for developing breast cancer.*

D. The International Breast Intervention Study I (IBIS I)[12]

1. *The study closely replicated the findings in BCPT.*
2. *In IBIS I, more than 7,000 women aged 35 to 70 years (median 50.7 years) at a high risk of breast cancer were randomly assigned to tamoxifen or placebo.*
3. *The primary endpoint was the incidence of breast cancer including ductal carcinoma in situ (DCIS).*
4. *Among the patients randomized, 3,574 received placebo and 3,578 received tamoxifen.*
5. *The median follow-up was 50 months, and the estimated compliance at five years was 77% among women in the placebo group and 67% among women taking tamoxifen.*
6. *The women in the study had a fourfold increased risk of developing breast cancer compared with the usual population, in most cases because of family history.*
7. *The overall reduction in the risk of developing breast cancer when comparing women taking tamoxifen to those taking placebo was 32%.*
8. *Among women who took HRT during the trial, the reduction in the incidence of breast cancer was 27% as compared with 26% among women who had never taken HRT.*
9. *The reduction in breast cancer incidence associated with tamoxifen was independent of age, and there was no difference between tamoxifen and placebo cases in nodal status, size, or grade of breast cancers diagnosed.*

TABLE 7.1	Risks and Benefits of SERMS		
	HRT	**Tamoxifen**	**Raloxifene**
Breast cancer	↑	↓	?
Total cholesterol	↓	↓	↓
Cardiovascular disease risk	↑	?	?
Bone mineral density	↑	↑	↑
Thrombotic events	↑	↑	↑
Menopausal symptoms	↓	↑	↑

Hayes, DF. Atlas of Breast Cancer. 2nd ed. London: Mosby; 2000

V. **Summary Benefits versus Risks of SERMs (Table 7.1)**[13,14]

  A. Most reported effects are associated with tamoxifen; raloxifene and other agents are not as extensively studied.

  B. Effects on bone density.

   1. *Many other agents are in clinical trials at the present time.*

   2. *In postmenopausal women, tamoxifen appears to prevent bone loss.*

   3. *In premenopausal women, tamoxifen results in a slight reduction in bone mineral density.*[8]

  C. Cardiovascular effects.

   1. *Total cholesterol levels are reduced significantly.*

   2. *Reduction in LDL cholesterol can be seen as early as two months after initiation of therapy with tamoxifen.*

   3. *Fibrinogen, homocysteine, and lipoprotein levels are reduced.*

  D. Gynecological effects.[8,9,15]

   1. *Premenopausal women may or may not note irregular menstrual cycles; pregnancy is possible.*

   2. *Postmenopausal women are at increased risk of uterine lining proliferation resulting in increased risk of endometrial carcinoma. Any vaginal spotting should be evaluated. Screening with yearly pap smear recommended with transvaginal ultrasound (TVUS) indicated only for evaluation of signs/symptoms. Screening with TVUS not found to be beneficial.*

   3. *All endometrial cancers from the BCPT were FIGO stage I, with all remaining cured except for one woman who was on the placebo arm and declined gynecologic intervention and ultimately died.*

   4. *In the BCPT, there was no increase in uterine cancer in women under 50 when analyzed by age group.*

   5. *Data from the BCPT indicates that endometrial cancer appears to be a concern for women over the age of 65.*

   6. *The longer a woman takes tamoxifen, the greater her risk for endometrial cancer with continued risk following cessation of the drug.*

   7. *The three-year actuarial endometrial cancer-specific survival was significantly worse for long-term users than for nonusers.*

   8. *Endometrial tumors in tamoxifen-treated women were associated with a worse survival.*

9. Women taking tamoxifen for five years or greater and developing endometrial cancer had tumors that were often P53 positive and more often had negative estrogen receptor levels than those of nonusers.

E. Sixty percent of women randomized to the tamoxifen arm of the BCPT experienced hot flashes.

F. Clotting events.

1. BCPT clotting events were not significantly increased in younger women.

2. In postmenopausal women over the age of 50, risk of pulmonary embolus and deep vein thrombosis is increased by threefold.

G. Cataract development.[16]

1. The Tamoxifen Opthalmic Evaluation Study (TOES)

a. Main objective was to estimate the prevalence of adverse changes in visual function and ocular structures associated with long-term use of tamoxifen.

i. Three hundred three women stratified into one of three groups: no history of prior tamoxifen use; tamoxifen use for an average of 4.8 years; and tamoxifen use for an average of 7.8 years.

ii. No difference noted in those without history of tamoxifen use compared with either group with history of tamoxifen use regarding:

- Visual function—daily visual function, visual acuities, contrast sensitivity
- Ocular structures—corneal opacities, lens opacities, macular edema, optic nerve abnormalities

iii. Differences were observed between the women who took tamoxifen and the women not taking tamoxifen regarding:

- Posterior subcapsular opacities
- Color confusion
- Intraretinal crystals
- Nausea

VI. **Recommendations on the Use of Tamoxifen and Raloxifene for Risk Reduction (Table 7.2)**

A. The American Society of Clinical Oncology (ASCO) conducted an evidence-based assessment of chemoprevention interventions available to reduce the incidence of developing invasive breast cancer.[17]

1. Outcomes of interest included breast cancer incidence, breast cancer-specific survival, overall survival, and the net health benefit of the interventions.

2. A comprehensive, formal literature review was conducted for the relevant topics, and testimony was collected from invited experts and interested parties following the ASCO-prescribed technology assessment procedure. More weight was given to published randomized trials than to other forms of evidence.

3. The ASCO Cancer Technology Assessment Working Group concluded that for women with a defined 5-year projected breast cancer risk of > 1.66%, tamoxifen 20 mg daily for five years may be offered to reduce their risk.

TABLE 7.2	Using Tamoxifen for the Reduction of Breast Cancer Risk

Women in whom tamoxifen should be considered:

- History of lobular carcinoma in situ (LCIS)
- History of ductal carcinoma in situ (DCIS)
- History of atypical ductal or lobular hyperplasia
- Premenopausal women with mutations in either the BRCA1 or BRCA2 genes or other predisposing genetic mutations
- Premenopausal women with 5-year probability of breast cancer ≥ 1.7% as determined using multivariable risk model predictions

Women in whom caution should be used when considering the use of tamoxifen:

- History of stroke, transient ischemic attack, deep vein thrombosis, and pulmonary embolus
- History of cataracts or cataract surgery
- Current use of hormone replacement therapy

Women who may consider the use of tamoxifen:

- Remote history of estrogen receptor-positive invasive breast cancer with no history of adjuvant tamoxifen therapy
- Postmenopausal women with osteoporosis and increased risk of breast cancer (These women should consider participation in the STAR trial.)

Modified from Vogel VG. Chemoprevention: reducing breast cancer risk, in Vogel VG, ed. *Management of Patients at High Risk for Breast Cancer.* Malden, MA: Blackwell Science, Inc. 2001;201–227. Used with permission of the publisher.

4. *Risk/benefit models suggest that the greatest clinical benefit with the least side effects is derived from use of tamoxifen in younger (premenopausal) women who are less likely to have thromboembolic sequelae and uterine cancer, in women without a uterus, and in women at higher risk for breast cancer.*

5. *Available data do not yet suggest that tamoxifen provides an overall health benefit or increases survival, although survival was not an intended outcome of the completed studies.*

6. *ASCO recommended that in all circumstances, tamoxifen use should be discussed as part of an informed decision-making process with careful consideration of individually calculated risks and benefits.*

7. *Use of tamoxifen combined with hormone replacement therapy, use of raloxifene, any aromatase inhibitor or inactivator, or fenretinide to lower the risk of developing breast cancer was not recommended outside the setting of a clinical trial.*

B. The U.S. Preventive Services Task Force (USPSTF) evaluated the strategies that are available for the primary prevention of breast cancer.[18,19]

1. *Their recommendations were slightly more conservative than ASCO's and addressed issues relevant to entire populations of women rather than only women with specific risk factors.*

2. The USPSTF recommended against the routine use of tamoxifen or raloxifene for the primary prevention of breast cancer in women at low or average risk for breast cancer.

3. The USPSTF found "fair evidence that tamoxifen and raloxifene may prevent some breast cancers in women at low or average risk for breast cancer, based on extrapolation from studies of women at higher risk."

4. They concluded, however, that the potential harms of chemoprevention may outweigh the potential benefits in women who are not at high risk for breast cancer.

5. The task force found fair evidence that treatment with tamoxifen can significantly reduce the risk for invasive estrogen-receptor-positive breast cancer in women at high risk for breast cancer and that the likelihood of benefit increases as the risk for breast cancer increases.

6. They found consistent but less abundant evidence for the benefit of raloxifene.

7. They also found good evidence that tamoxifen and raloxifene increase the risk for thromboembolic events (for example, stroke, pulmonary embolism, and deep venous thrombosis) and symptomatic side effects and that tamoxifen (but not raloxifene) increases the risk for endometrial cancer.

8. The task force concluded that the balance of benefits and harms may be favorable for some high-risk women but will depend on breast cancer risk, risk for potential harms, and individual patient preferences.

9. They recommended that clinicians discuss chemoprevention with women at high risk for breast cancer and at low risk for adverse effects of chemoprevention, and they indicated that clinicians should inform patients of the potential benefits and harms of chemoprevention.

VII. **Management of SERM-related Side Effects (see also Chapter 8)**
   A. Hot flashes
      1. Hot flashes are caused by a diminished level of estrogen with a direct effect on the hypothalamus (part of the brain that regulates appetite, sleep cycles, sex hormones, and body temperature) causing it to read "too hot," making the brain communicate to other parts of the body to get rid of the heat.
      2. This leads to the heart pumping faster and cutaneous blood vessels dilating to circulate more blood to radiate heat.
      3. Sweat glands release sweat to cool the body.
   B. It may take 4 to 6 weeks for some of these interventions to work. Instructions for patients:
      1. Absorbent cotton, linen, or rayon clothing instead of wool, synthetics, or silk is recommended.
      2. Avoid turtlenecks.
      3. Use cotton sheets.
      4. Take a cool shower prior to going to bed.
      5. Keep ice water on hand to sip to cool down.

6. *Dress in layers.*
7. *Lower the thermostat.*
8. *Avoid caffeine and spicy foods.*
9. *Exercise regularly.*
10. *Identify the triggers for your hot flashes.*
11. *Minimize stress.*
12. *Reduce alcohol consumption.*
13. *Avoid diet pills.*
14. *Avoid saunas, hot showers, and hot tubs.*
15. *Cool yourself off during hot weather.*
16. *Reduce or stop smoking.*
17. *Reduce caffeine consumption.*
18. *Practice relaxation techniques.*
19. *Keep a journal of the hot flashes with number and times of occurrence.*
20. *Take Vitamin B complex with meals.*
21. *Take Vitamin E.*
22. *Take 800 IU of Vitamin E PO daily—available over the counter.*
23. *Take Clonidine.*
    a. 0.1 mg patch weekly—prescription required
    b. 0.1–0.2 mg tablet daily or twice per day—prescription required
24. *Take Venlafaxine hydrochloride (Effexor®).*
    a. 37.5 mg tablet one or two daily at night—prescription required.
    b. Recent clinical trial recommended the use of at least 75 mg for effectiveness.
25. *Phenobarbital-belladonna-ergotamine combination (Bellergal-S).*
    a. One tablet at night—prescription required
26. *Paroxetine hydrochloride (Paxil).*
    a. One 10 mg tablet daily for one week then increase to one 20 mg tablet daily—prescription required
27. *Phytoestrogens.*
    a. They are found in food products such as soy. They help with hot flashes but are not encouraged for women with an increased risk for developing breast cancer.
    b. A 12-week study of 145 menopausal women in Israel found that 78 women assigned to a phytoestrogen-rich (tofu, soy drink, miso, ground flaxseed) diet had significantly fewer hot flashes and vaginal dryness than the 36 women in the control group that maintained their normal diet.[20]
28. *Acupuncture: a group treated with standard acupuncture had 50% reduction in number of hot flashes and sustained benefit greater than three months after treatment.*[21]
29. *Dong quai/angelica sinensis.*[22]
    a. Seventy-one postmenopasual women experiencing hot flashes were randomized to receive either dong quai or placebo. After 24 weeks, no statistically significant differences were noted between groups.
    b. Dong quai contains psoralens, which can cause photosensitization and dermatitis.

30. Evening primrose oil.[23]
    a. A randomized double-blind study of GLA to treat vasomotor symptoms during menopause found that women taking GLA reported significant improvement in the number of nighttime hot flashes.
    b. Evening primrose oil contains gamma linolenic acid.
31. Black cohosh/cimicifuga racemosa.[24]
    a. Eight studies on black cohosh conducted over the past four decades conclude that black cohosh selectively suppresses LH with no effect on FSH.
    b. The German Commission E has approved the use of black cohosh for menopausal symptoms but recommends limiting its use to six months.
    c. There are no known contraindications.
C. Vaginal dryness—instructions for patients:
   1. Take warm baths to alleviate vaginal itching and discomfort.
   2. Wear cotton underwear.
   3. Avoid:
      a. Douches
      b. Feminine hygiene spray
      c. Perfumed soaps
      d. Perfumed toilet paper
      e. Scented fabric softener
      f. Scented dryer sheets
   4. Use water-based moisturizers/lubricants such as Replens, Astroglide, Gyne-Moistrin, Lubrin vaginal suppositories, and other over-the-counter moisturizers/lubricants.
   5. Take acidophilus capsules, which are available over the counter.
   6. Take one 460 mg acidophilus capsule by mouth daily.
   7. Discuss with your gynecologist use of an Estring® (Pfizer).
      a. Available by prescription from gynecologist as an estrogen-filled ring inserted by the individual into the upper third of the vagina, much like a diaphragm, worn continuously with replacements every three months
      b. Exerts hormonal effects locally and only detectable systemically in the first 24 hours
      c. Approved for women with breast cancer on clinical trials
      d. Especially helpful for young women made prematurely postmenopausal either surgically or chemically where vaginal dryness is severe and/or prolonged
   8. Take zinc tablets.
      a. Take one 15-mg tablet by mouth daily
      b. Apply Vitamin E oil topically to help hydrate the vaginal membrane
      c. Vitamin E suppositories available for insertion
   9. Try Vagifem®.
      a. This treatment is available by prescription.
      b. This treatment contains low-dose, slow-release vaginal matrix tablet containing 25 ug of 17 beta-estradiol.
      c. Vagifem is the only vaginal tablet available containing estrogen derived from plants.
      d. 17 beta-estradiol is identical to the estrogen produced in a woman's body prior to menopause.

  e. Insert one tablet into the vagina nightly for two weeks and then one tablet vaginally twice weekly.
  f. Vagifem delivers the estrogen directly to the vagina.
  g. One may not notice improvement for up to two weeks.
  h. This treatment is well tolerated with minimal systemic absorption.
  i. Use cautiously with a history of endometrial hyperplasia or gallbladder disease.

10. *Try intravaginal yogurt.*
  a. Use plain live culture yogurt.
  b. Apply yogurt intravaginally with a baby bulb syringe every night for seven nights.
  c. After the seven nights, apply yogurt three times per week for an additional three weeks.
  d. The same day you begin the intravaginal yogurt also start to eat live culture yogurt on a regular basis.
  e. Once you have completed the course of intravaginal yogurt, continue to eat yogurt daily to maintain your comfort level.

VIII. New and Promising Agents for Breast Cancer Risk Reduction

A. Aromatase inhibitor anastrozole (Arimidex®) has shown to be superior to tamoxifen for the adjuvant treatment of breast cancer in postmenopausal women with an improvement in disease-free survival.

1. *Mechanism of action: Arimidex is a nonsteroidal aromatase inhibitor that lowers the amount of circulating estrogens by stopping the production of estrogen in adipose tissue, the main source of estrogen in postmenopausal women.*

2. *ATAC Trial (Arimidex versus Tamoxifen Alone or in Combination as Adjuvant Therapy in Postmenopausal Women with Early Breast Cancer).*[25]
  a. There were fewer contralateral breast cancers and less toxicity.
  b. Other aromatase inhibitors continue evaluation in clinical trials for adjuvant treatment recommendations and comparisons.
  c. Risk of both arthralgias and fractures is more common with anastrozole compared with tamoxifen. A bone density test is recommended prior to initiation to assess osteopenia or osteoporosis.
  d. The trial randomized 9,366 postmenopausal women in 21 countries from July 1996 to March 2000, with approximately 3,100 per arm.
  e. Preliminary results after 2.5 years were released in San Antonio in December 2001.
  f. No additional benefit was noted in the combination arm when compared with tamoxifen alone.
  g. This treatment is *not* to be used in premenopausal women.
  h. Dosage: 1 mg daily, orally.
  i. The side effects, when compared with tamoxifen, show significantly fewer reports of:
      i. Endometrial cancer (0.5% versus 1%)
      ii. Deep vein thrombosis (1% versus 1.7%)
      iii. Stroke (1% versus 2.1%)

      iv. Hot flashes (34.3% versus 39.7%)

      v. Arimidex was associated with more fractures (5.8% versus 3.7% compared with tamoxifen).

3. *Indication: may be more beneficial with postmenopausal women with a history of thromboembolic events, uterine bleeding on tamoxifen, or severe side effects while on tamoxifen.*

4. *No aromatase inhibitor is yet approved by FDA for the reduction of breast cancer risk.*

5. *Study of Tamoxifen and Raloxifene (STAR) trial.*

    a. This is a national trial with over 500 centers across the United States and Canada being coordinated by the NSABP (National Surgical Adjuvant Breast and Bowel Project).

    b. The primary goal of the trial is to determine which drug, tamoxifen (Nolvadex®) or raloxifene (Evista®), will be more effective in lowering the incidence of breast cancer in postmenopausal women with an increased risk with fewer side effects.

    c. Risk is calculated using the Gail model.

    d. The accrual goal is 22,000 women nationally with the enrollment period being for five years, having started in July 1999.

    e. At the time of this writing, there are more than 14,000 women enrolled with a target accrual of 22,000 subjects.

    f. The trial is designed with a multistep entry process to encourage compliance and eliminate the women who are not going to be dedicated to comply with the trial for seven years.

    g. The trial is a double-blind design with two arms.

    h. Women are randomized to take either tamoxifen 20 mg per day and a placebo that looks like raloxifene or raloxifene 60 mg per day and a placebo that looks like tamoxifen for five years.

    i. Participants will take their study drug for five years and be followed for seven years, possibly longer, to evaluate any long-term side effects associated with tamoxifen or raloxifene use.

    j. There are three main eligibility criteria for the STAR trial:

      i. Women must be postmenopausal.

      ii. Women must be at least 35 years of age.

      iii. Women must have an increased risk for breast cancer determined utilizing the Gail Model.

    k. Required follow-up exams include:

      i. Obtaining annual bilateral mammograms

      ii. Annual bimanual pelvic exams unless the woman has had a total abdominal hysterectomy and bilateral salpingo-oophorectomy

      iii. Breast exams every six months by a medical professional

      iv. Physical exam annually

      v. A complete blood count with platelets and chemistry panel annually

B. Toremifene citrate (Fareston®).

  1. *Mechanism of action*

  2. *Indicated for postmenopausal women in the metastatic setting with ER positive tumors as an alternative first line agent*

  3. *Not approved for chemoprevention*

4. *Nonsteroidal antiestrogen binds to the estrogen receptor*

5. *Dosage: 60 mg, once daily, orally*

6. *Side effects*

   a. Similar to tamoxifen including hot flashes, night sweats, nausea, vaginal discharge, edema, vomiting, and vaginal bleeding

   b. May try as an alternative if not able to tolerate tamoxifen due to hot flashes, edema, or nausea

   c. Vaginal bleeding reported

7. *Not enough data yet to determine Fareston's role in either treatment or risk reduction*

IX. Alternative Agents

A. Indole-3-Carbinol

   1. *Dosage: One capsule twice per day orally for women under 120 pounds; for 120–180 pounds, one capsule three times per day*

   2. *Each capsule contains 200 mg indole-3-carbinol*

   3. *Increases the conversion of estradiol to 2-OH estrogen and decreases production of 16-OH estrogen, which has been shown to reduce breast cancer incidence*

   4. *Stops human cancer cells from growing and provokes the cells to self-destruct (apoptosis)*

   5. *Not yet approved for breast cancer risk reduction*

B. Omega-3 polyunsaturated fatty acids

C. Antioxidants

X. Chemoprevention for patients with BRCA1/BRCA2 mutations[26]

A. There are no prospective data available on use of chemoprevention and risk reduction in mutation carriers.

B. Carriers are at high risk for development of both breast and ovarian cancer.

C. BRCA1 acts in part as a tumor suppressor gene with reduction in BRCA1 expression leading to an increase in development of breast and ovarian cell lines with overexpression causing a delay in growth.

   1. *Both BRCA1 and BRCA2 seem to be regulated by common pathways.*

   2. *Expression of both genes is differentially regulated by hormones during the development of specific target tissues, but the upregulation of mRNA expression in the breast by ovarian steroid hormones is greater for BRCA1 than for BRCA2.*

   3. *Women carrying a BRCA1 mutation are more likely to develop ER negative tumors, but with a prophylactic oophorectomy, women carrying BRCA1 or BRCA2 mutations can reduce their risk of developing breast cancer by approximately 30 to 50%.*

D. Tamoxifen may be appropriate to offer to mutation carriers to reduce the risk of breast cancer with appropriate informed consent.

XI. Ethical Issues
   A. Timing of chemoprevention.
   B. Best age for initiation is not determined.
   C. Risk of breast cancer rises with age.
   D. Discussion with patient is important to optimize timing.

XII. Breast Cancer Prevention Information
   A. Weber ES. Questions & answers about breast cancer diagnosis. *Am J Nurs* 1997;97:34–38.
   B. National Cancer Institute Information Service 1-800-4-CANCER (1-800-422-6237)
   C. National Alliance of Breast Cancer Organizations 212-719-0154
   D. American Cancer Society 1-800-227-2345
   E. Susan G. Komen Breast Cancer Foundation 1-800-462-9273
   F. Y-ME 1-800-221-2141 (9AM to 5PM CSF) or 312-986-8228 (24 hours)
   G. http://cancernet.nci.nih.gov—to reach the NCI's risk assessment web site
   H. http://oncolink.upenn.edu/ (University of Pennsylvania web site)
   I. Cancer Fax—fax on demand service at 1-800-624-2511
   J. http://www.breastcancerprevention.org

References
1. Vogel VG. Chemoprevention: reducing breast cancer risk. In: Vogel VG, ed. *Management of Patients at High Risk for Breast Cancer.* Malden, MA: Blackwell Science Inc; 2001:201–227.

2. *CIG Fact Sheet* NCI.

3. Gail MH, Brinton LA, Byar DP, et al. Projecting individualized probabilities of developing breast cancer for white females who are being examined annually. *J Natl Cancer Inst* 1989;81:1879–1886.

4. Fisher B, Costantino JP, Wickerham DL, et al. Tamoxifen for prevention of breast cancer: Report of the National Surgical Adjuvant Breast and Bowel Project P-1 Study. *J Natl Cancer Inst* 1998;90:1371–1388.

5. Cummings SR, Eckert S, Krueger KA, et al. The effect of raloxifene on risk of breast cancer in postmenopausal women: results from the MORE randomized trial. *JAMA* 1999;281:2189–2197.

6. Lippman ME, Krueger KA, Eckert S, et al. Indicators of lifetime estrogen exposure: effect on breast cancer incidence and interaction with raloxifene therapy in the multiple outcomes of raloxifene evaluation study participants. *J Clin Oncol* 2001;19:3111–3116.

7. Pritchard KI. Selective estrogen receptor modulators in the prevention and treatment of breast cancer. *Clinical Oncology Updates* 2001;3:1–15.

8. O'Regan RM, Gradishar WJ. Selective estrogen receptor modulators in 2001. *Oncology* 2001;15:1177–1194.

9. Day R, Ganz PA, Costantino JP, et al. Health-related quality of life and tamoxifen in breast cancer prevention: a report from the National Surgical Adjuvant Breast and Bowel Project P-1 Study. *J Clin Oncol* 1999;17:2659–2669.

10. Powles TJ. The Royal Marsden Hospital (RMH) trial: key points and remaining questions. *Ann New York Acad Sci* 2001;949:109–112.

11. Veronesi U, Maisonneuve P, Sacchini V, Rotmensz N, Boyle P. Italian Tamoxifen Study Group. Tamoxifen for breast cancer among hysterectomised women. *Lancet* 2002;359:1122–1124.

12. Cuzick J, Forbes J, Edwards R, et al. First results from the International Breast Cancer Intervention Study (IBIS-1): a randomized prevention trial. *Lancet* 2002; 360:817–824.

13. Hayes DF. *Atlas of Breast Cancer*, 2nd ed. Mosby; 2000.

14. Gail MH, Costantino JP, Bryant J, et al. Weighing the risks and benefits of tamoxifen treatment for preventing breast cancer. *J Natl Cancer Inst* 1999;91:1829–1846.

15. Bergman L, Beelen ML, Gallee MP, et al. Risk and prognosis of endometrial cancer after tamoxifen for breast cancer. Comprehensive Cancer Centres' ALERT Group. Assessment of Liver and Endometrial Cancer Risk following Tamoxifen. *Lancet* 2000;356:881–887.

16. Gorin MB, Day R, Costantino JP, et al. Long-term tamoxifen citrate use and potential ocular toxicity. *Amer J Ophthalmol* 1998;125:493–501.

17. Chlebowski R, Col N, Weiner E, et al., for the ASCO Breast Cancer Technology Assessment Working Group. American Society of Clinical Oncology technology assessment of pharmacologic interventions for breast cancer risk reduction including tamoxifen, raloxifene, and aromatase inhibition. *J Clin Oncol* 2002;20:3328–2243.

18. Kinsinger LS, Harris R, Woolf SH, et al. Chemoprevention of breast cancer: A summary of the evidence for the U.S. Preventive Services Task Force. *Ann Intern Med* 2002;137:59–67.

19. US Preventive Services Task Force. Chemoprevention of breast cancer: recommendation and rationale. *Ann Intern Med.* 2002;137:56–58.

20. Brezinski A, et al. Short-term effects of phytoestrogen-rich diet on postmenopausal women. *Menopause* 1997;4:89–94.

21. Wyon Y, Lindgren R, Hammar M, et al. Acupuncture against climacteric disorders? Lower number of symptoms after menopause. *Lakartidningen* 1994;91:2318–2322.

22. Hirata JD, Swiersz LM, Zell B, et al. Does dong quai have estrogenic effects in postmenopausal? A double-blind, placebo controlled trial. *Fertil Sterility* 1997;68:981–986.

23. Chenoy R, Hussain S, et al. Effect of oral gamma linolenic acid from evening primrose oil on menopausal flushing. *BMJ* 1994;308:501–503.

24. Lieberman S. A review of the effectiveness of black cohosh for the symptoms of menopause. *J Womens Health* 1998;7:525–529.

25. The ATAC (Arimidex, Tamoxifen Alone or in Combination) Trialists' Group. Anastrozole alone or in combination with tamoxifen versus tamoxifen alone for adjuvant treatment of postmenopausal women with early breast cancer: first results of the ATAC randomised trial. *Lancet* 2002;359:2131–2139.

26. Vogel VG. Reducing the risk of breast cancer with tamoxifen in women at increased risk. *J Clin Oncol* 2001;19:87s–92s.

Hormone Replacement Therapy

Marita V. Lazzaro, MS, RN, CS-ANP
Adult and Women's Health Nurse Practitioner
Cancer Prevention Center
The University of Texas M. D. Anderson Cancer Center
Houston, TX

Therese Bevers, MD
Medical Director
Cancer Prevention Center
The University of Texas M. D. Anderson Cancer Center
Houston, TX

chapter 8

Evidence-Based Risks and Benefits of Hormone Replacement Therapy (HRT)

The majority of women do experience some degree of menopausal symptoms, and approximately 35 to 38% of postmenopausal women in the United States are using HRT (either estrogen alone or in combination with progesterone).[1] There is confusion regarding the safety of HRT and widespread interest in natural and alternative therapies. Reported research studies now provide evidence-based data on HRT and its alternatives. With this new information regarding the risks and benefits of HRT, patients will need guidance to make informed decisions regarding conventional hormone therapy, the more recently developed "designer estrogens" (i.e., the selective estrogen receptor modulators raloxifene or tamoxifen), and alternative or complementary therapies.

Women will not often broach the subject of HRT with their clinicians. It is incumbent upon the clinician to address these issues of menopause and the benefits and risks of available interventions with all perimenopausal and postmenopausal patients.

I. **Menopause**
    A. Definition: Menopause is marked as the permanent cessation of reproductive function and defined as the cessation of menstrual cycles for one full year.
        1. *Natural menopause is a physiological event that occurs in 100% of aging women.*
            a. Associated with a decrease in the circulating estrogen as the causative factor. After menopause, circulating estradiol concentration is about one-half of the concentration prior to menopause and is mostly a product of peripheral conversion of androgen to estrone.
            b. Natural menopause occurs most commonly in the late fifth and early sixth decade as ovarian function declines and ceases.
            c. The average age of menopause in the United States is 51 years.
            d. Menopausal symptoms may be experienced up to five years prior to the cessation of menstruation. This is considered the perimenopausal state and, on average, occurs around 45 to 47 years of age.
            e. The sixth decade is also associated with an increased risk of cardiovascular disease, cancer, osteoporosis, psychological stress, cognitive decline, and Alzheimer's disease.
        2. *Surgical menopause occurs with the surgical removal of both ovaries, with or without the uterus.*
        3. *Clinical menopause occurs when medical treatment of a disease results in the permanent cessation of ovarian function.*
        4. *Menopause can be accompanied by classic symptoms experienced to some degree by 85 to 90% of all women.*
            a. The endocrine changes of menopause are permanent.
            b. Some of the classic symptoms can decrease over time.

    c. Others, such as the majority of urogenital problems, may increase over time.

B. Etiology: Estrogens are largely responsible for the development and maintenance of the female reproductive system.

   1. *Circulating estradiol, estrone, and estriol exist in a dynamic equilibrium.*

   2. *Estradiol, produced by the ovaries, is the principal intracellular estrogen and is more potent at the estrogen receptor than its metabolites.*

   3. *Estrogen receptors are found in the female reproductive organs, breasts, pituitary, hypothalamus, liver, bone, and cardiovascular system.*

   4. *Estrogen concentration modulates the pituitary secretion of the gonadotrophins, luteinizing hormone (LH) and follicle-stimulating hormone (FSH), through a negative feedback mechanism.*

   5. *In an ovulating female, the ovarian follicle secretes 70–500 ug of estradiol daily (depending on the cycle phase). This ceases with the onset of menopause.*

   6. *Postmenopausally, estrone and estrone sulfate are the primary circulating estrogens, produced in the peripheral tissues through the conversion of androstenedione from the adrenal cortex, about 45 ug/24 hours.*

C. Evidence-based impact of hormone therapy.

   1. *Previously available information was based on observational studies regarding hormone replacement therapy and cardiovascular disease, osteoporosis, and quality of life issues.*

     a. The majority of these studies showed positive effects.

     b. Benefits may be influenced by differences in educational levels, cultural beliefs, access to medical care, lifestyles, and compliance with management recommendations of those seeking HRT.[1]

   2. *Four randomized studies address the effect of HRT on lipoproteins and primary and secondary prevention of cardiovascular disease in women with and without coronary heart disease.*

     a. The Postmenopausal Estrogen/Progestin Interventions (PEPI) Trial[2]

     b. The Heart and Estrogen/Progestin Replacement Study (HERS)[3]

     c. The Estrogen Replacement and Atherosclerosis Trial (ERA)[4]

     d. The Papworth Hormone-Replacement Therapy Atherosclerosis Study[5]

   3. *Two ongoing, large-scale, randomized studies will provide information on the risks and benefits of HRT on medical, psychological, and quality of life issues.*

     a. The Women's Health Initiative in the United States[6]

     b. The Women's International Study of Long Duration Oestrogen after Menopause in 14 countries (results in 2012)[7]

   4. *Evidence of HRT can be categorized into definite benefits, definite risks, probable risks, and risks and benefits needing further investigation (Table 8.1).*[1]

TABLE 8.1	Benefits and Risks of Postmenopausal Hormone-Replacement Therapy (HRT)
Variable	Effect
Definite benefits	
Symptoms of menopause	Definite improvement
Osteoporosis	Definite increase in bone mineral density; probable decrease in risk of fractures
Definite risks	
Endometrial cancer	Definite increase in risk with use of unopposed estrogen; no increase with use of estrogen plus progestin
Venous thromboembolism	Definite increase in risk
Breast cancer	Definite increase in risk with use >2 yr
Probable increase in risk	
Gallbladder disease	Probable increase in risk

Benefit or Risk		Source of Data
Relative	**Absolute**	
>70-80% decrease		Observational studies and randomized trials*
2–5% increase in bone density; 25–50% decrease in risk of fractures	172 fewer hip fractures (402 versus 574) per 100,000 woman-years	Observational studies and limited data from randomized trials*
Increase in risk by a factor of 8 to 10 with use of unopposed estrogen** for >10 years; no excess risk with combined estrogen progestin	Excess of 46 cases (52 versus 6) per 100,000 woman-years of unopposed estrogen use (>10 yr of use); no excess with use of combined therapy	Observational studies and randomized trials*
Increase in risk by a factor of 2.7	Secondary prevention: excess of 390 cases per 100,000 woman-years	Heart and Estrogen/Progestin Replacement Study
	Primary prevention: excess of 20 cases per 100,000 woman-years	Observational studies
Overall increase in risk by a factor of 1.26–1.35 with HRT use >2 years	Excess of 20 cases per 10,000 women using HRT for 5 years; 60 excess cases after 10 years of use; 120 excess cases after 15 years of use	Meta-analysis of 51 observational studies; Women's Health Initiative
Increase in risk by a factor of 1.4	Excess of 360 cases per 100,000 woman-years	Heart and Estrogen/Progestin Replacement Study

continued on page 104

TABLE 8.1 CONTINUED	Benefits and Risks of Postmenopausal Hormone-Replacement Therapy (HRT)
Variable	**Effect**
Uncertain benefits and risks	
Cardiovascular disease Primary prevention	Probable net harm
Secondary prevention	Probable early increase in risk
Colorectal cancer	Possible but unproven decrease in risk
Cognitive dysfunction	Unproven decrease in risk (inconsistent results)

* *Observational data suggest a decrease in risk of 35 to 50%, whereas randomized trial data show no effect or a possible harmful effect during the first one or two years of use. Most studies have accessed conjugated equine estrogen alone or in combination with medroxyprogesterone acetate.*

** *The term "unopposed estrogen" refers to the use of estrogen without medroxyprogesterone acetate.*

Reproduced by permission from Manson J, Martin K. Postmenopausal hormone replacement therapy. *N Engl J Med* 2001;345:34–40.

 5. *Randomized studies have provided definitive evidence on the positive effects of HRT on osteoporosis prevention.*[1]

II. **Definite Benefits of HRT**
   A. Quality of life issues: In a Scottish survey of 6,096 women aged 45 to 54 years, 84% of the women experienced at least one classic menopausal symptom, with 45% experiencing two or more.[1] Randomized and observational studies confirm the positive benefits of HRT on classic symptoms.

   1. *Classic menopausal symptoms: Thyroid disorders and depression can mimic these symptoms and need to be included in the differential diagnosis.*
      a. Vasodilation symptoms: Estrogen receptors serve as a transcription factor regulating vasomotor tone.
         i. Lack of estrogen acts on the hypothalamus to trigger vasodilation for "perceived" body temperature control that is physiologically unnecessary.
         ii. Occurs to some extent in 80 to 85% of menopausal women and is the most common complaint of perimenopausal and early menopause; 10 to 15% of these women experience severe symptoms.[6]
         iii. Symptoms usually decrease over time, with resolution within two years of menopause in 70% of women.

Benefit or Risk		Source of Data
Relative	Absolute	
Uncertain	Uncertain	Observational studies and randomized trials*
Uncertain	Uncertain	Observational studies and randomized trials*
20% decrease	24 fewer cases (96 versus120) per 100,000 woman-years	Observational studies
Uncertain	Uncertain	Observational studies and randomized trials*

    iv. Symptoms can be exacerbated by "triggers" including stress, smoking, and temperature changes (i.e., hot showers, saunas, and certain foods, including caffeine, alcohol, diet pills, and spicy foods).

    v. Estrone is a natural estrogen produced in fat and muscle; heavier or more muscular women may experience fewer symptoms than thin women.

    vi. Symptoms respond well to lifestyle changes, medication, alternative therapies, and time.

  b. Urogenital symptoms.

    i. Vaginal dryness with associated mild to moderate vaginal atrophy occurs in 85 to 90% of women.[6] Severe atrophy occurs in only 10 to 15% of women.

    ii. These symptoms have a later onset of occurrence and increase over time. Some level of vaginal dryness is experienced within three years of menopause with more severe symptoms occurring five to ten years later.

    iii. Dyspareunia can accompany vaginal dryness and atrophy and can be severe enough to limit sexual activity. This is the major complaint expressed with vaginal changes and correlates with sexual activity, decreasing as activity decreases.

    iv. The occurrence of cystitis and urinary tract infections is aggravated by vaginal irritation. Vaginal dryness and atrophy combined with certain activities increases irritation. Activities include sexual activity, some exercises (especially those associated with tight clothing), and sports (i.e., horseback riding, bicycling, etc.).

    v. Resolution is best achieved with prescription medication. Over-the-counter medication can be an effective alternative in mild cases and as early prevention.

c. Mood swings.

    i. Moods swings are similar to those experienced with premenstrual syndrome (PMS), including irritability and emotional lability.

    ii. Triggers include stress and fatigue.

    iii. Symptoms occur mainly in perimenopausal and early menopause and decrease with time. Resolution is experienced in 50% of women within two to three years of menopause and in the majority of women by ten years.[6]

    iv. Depression should be ruled out if symptoms continue with adequate intervention, increase over time, or recur after initial resolution.

    v. Symptoms respond well to lifestyle changes, medication, complementary therapies, and time.

d. Decrease in sexual interest.

    i. Decreased libido with subsequent slowness in sexual response occurs to some extent in the majority of women. Onset usually occurs within the first two years of menopause, with symptoms leveling off thereafter.

    ii. Severe cases with inability to achieve orgasm are rare.

    iii. Underlying factors may contribute to decreased sexual interest including depression, fatigue secondary to sleep disturbances, and painful intercourse due to vaginal dryness and atrophy.

    iv. Medication associated with age-related chronic illnesses, such as diabetes mellitus, hypertension, and depression may be a contributing factor.

    v. Response is achieved with lifestyle changes (especially stress reduction, exercise, and counseling with the partner). Less than 50% improvement occurs with medication alone.

    vi. Studies involving low-dose testosterone therapy are ongoing.

e. Sleep disturbances may be experienced as interruptions due to night sweats, inability to achieve sleep or stay asleep, and vivid dreams.

    i. These disturbances are experienced in fewer than 40 to 60% of postmenopausal women. Severe cases of true insomnia are seen in less than 10% of women.[6]

    ii. Depression and fatigue can be contributing factors.

    iii. Responds well to lifestyle changes, although a mild sleep aid may be needed in some cases. Contributing factors need to be managed separately.

2. *Prescriptive therapeutic interventions.*

a. There is excellent overall response to HRT, with a greater than 90% response in treated women. Estrogen vaginal inserts specifically target urogenital symptoms.

b. Some selective seratonin reuptake inhibitors (SSRIs) and mild sedatives show a positive impact on vasodilation symptoms, mood swings, and/or sleep disturbances.[8]

    i. Effexor XR®: 37.5 mg to 75 mg PO QD

    ii. Paxil CR®: 10 mg to 20 mg PO QD

    iii. Bellamine S: 1 tab PO QHS or BID

    c. Selected antihypertensives can control vasodilation symptoms.
       i. Clonidine: 0.1–0.4 mg/day PO divided BID/TID or
       ii. Clonidine: 0.1–0.3 mg/day transdermal patch
    d. Anecdotal information has shown positive effects of compounded natural estrogens in the relief of vasodilation symptoms, sleep disturbances, and mood swings. There are no controlled data from clinical trials.

3. *Nonprescriptive therapeutic interventions.*
    a. Studies are mainly observational and anecdotal.
    b. Vitamin E 800 IU/day has a positive effect on the vasodilation symptoms.[8]
    c. Periden-C (vitamin C and bioflavinoids) showed a positive impact on vasodilation symptoms in some observational studies.[8]
    d. While concentrated soy products have been shown to reduce vasodilation, mood swings, and vaginal dryness to some extent, no evidence-based studies regarding dosing and safety have been completed.
    e. Evening primrose oil, through observational studies for relief of PMS, has been reported to have positive effects on the vasodilation, mood swings, and sleep disturbances of menopause.
    f. Other complementary and herbal therapies such as black cohash, valaria, and kava kava require further study for definitive evidence on effectiveness, dosing, and safety.
    g. Water-soluble vaginal lubrications used on a regular basis can help alleviate vaginal dryness and slow the onset of vaginal atrophy (i.e., Astroglide, KY Jelly, Replens, Luprin, etc.).

4. *Lifestyle changes.*
    a. Sustained exercise of 30–40 minutes per day has a positive impact on all symptoms except urogenital ones. It should be recommended to some extent for all perimenopausal and menopausal women.
    b. Smoking increases vasodilation symptoms, which increases sleep disturbances; smoking cessation should be a part of all health programs. The process of smoking cessation may actually aggravate mood swings, and antidepressant therapy (e.g., Zyban®) should be considered.
    c. Nutritional interventions including phytoestrogens such as soy products, diets high in vitamins D, E, and B, and omega fatty acids may contribute to balanced mental and emotional health.
       i. Vitamin D 800 IU/day PO
       ii. Vitamin E 800 IU/day PO
       iii. Vitamin B complex 200 mg/day PO
    d. Avoidance of dietary triggers, such as caffeine, alcohol, diet pills, spicy foods, and hot foods, will decrease severity of vasodilation, mood swings, and sleep disturbances.
    e. Environmental control of temperature helps to reduce the severity of vasodilation symptoms.

B. Osteoporosis prevention.
  1. *Incidence and etiology.*
    a. In osteoporosis, bone mass is reduced, indicating that the rate of bone resorption exceeds the rate of bone formation.
    b. Type I osteoporosis is associated with menopause and presents with fractures involving the trabecular bones of the wrists, spine, and hips.[9]

  c. There is a 60% incidence of osteoporosis in menopausal women in the United States, with a significantly higher percentage of osteopenia.

  d. Approximately one-fourth of aging women sustain a vertebral or hip fracture between ages 60 and 90.[9]

  e. Calcium intake during the first three decades of life influences peak bone mass; calcium intake during adult life, however, continues to have a small positive effect.

  f. Interleukin 1 (IL1) stimulates production of interleukin 6 (IL6), which is the key cytokine in bone resorption in menopause. Circulating estrogen decreases IL1 and subsequently IL6, aiding in the prevention of osteoporosis.[9]

  g. Other risk factors include family history, lifelong history of poor dietary calcium intake, physical inactivity or immobilization, smoking, malnutrition, hypogonadal state, ingestion of high phosphate intake, (i.e., soft drinks, red meat, and caffeine [a calciuretic]). Lean body mass is associated with decreased adrenally produced estrone and is a risk factor especially in both Caucasian and Asian women.

2. *Prescriptive therapeutic interventions (Table 8.2)*[1]

  a. Clinical trials have shown a 25 to 50% reduction of bone loss and increase of bone density of the spine and hip with HRT in single or combination form.[1]

  b. Definitive evidence shows that bisphosphonates (e.g., Fosamax®) increase bone density of the spine, trochanter, and femoral neck and decrease fractures of the spine, hip, and nonvertebral bones by 50%.[1]

  c. Selective Estrogen Receptor Modulators, SERMs (i.e., tamoxifen and raloxifene).

   i. An increase in bone density of the spine and femoral neck and a reduction in vertebral fractures by 30% is shown in randomized studies.[8]

   ii. Raloxifene is FDA-approved for osteoporosis prevention.
- It probably decreases the risk of breast cancer, and is presently under study for this indication.[8]
- The safety of raloxifene in women with a personal history of breast cancer is unknown.

   iii. Tamoxifen is an alternative for women at increased risk for breast cancer.[8]
- The overall risk of breast cancer is reduced by 49%.
- Bone fractures are reduced.
- Cardiovascular benefits are uncertain.

   iv. SERMs may aggravate classic menopausal symptoms.

  d. Randomized studies of calcitonin show an increase in bone density.

   i. Limited studies show the beneficial effect is in treatment of osteoporosis rather than its prevention.

   ii. Efficacy decreases with long-term use, which may limit its effectiveness in prevention.[1]

3. *Nonprescriptive therapeutic interventions.*

  a. Although data from clinical trials are limited, calcium and vitamin D appear to preserve or increase bone density.[1]

   i. Calcium 1500 mg per day PO

   ii. Vitamin D 800 IU per day

| **TABLE 8.2** | Results of Randomized Clinical Trials of the Effectiveness of Therapies for Preventing or Treating Osteoporosis | | |

Therapy	Effect on Bone Mineral Density	Effect on Fractures	Comments
Hormone replacement therapy	Decreases rate of bone loss; increases bone density of the spine and hip	Decreases risk of vertebral fractures by approximately 50%; decreases risk of hip, wrist, and other nonvertebral fractures by 25–30%	Limited data from randomized trials; similar results with combination therapy, different regimens and routes of administration; benefits may be accentuated among women > 60 years old
Bisphosphonates (alendronate, risedronate)	Increases bone density of the spine, trochanter, and femoral neck	Decreases risk of vertebral, hip, and other nonvertebral fractures by 50%	May cause esophageal and gastrointestinal side effects
Selective estrogen receptor modulators (SERMs)	Increases bone density in the spine, and femoral neck	Reduces risk of new vertebral fractures by 30% among women with and without preexisting fractures; has no significant effect on nonvertebral fractures	May increase hot flashes; may increase the risk of venous thromboembolism; may lower the risk of breast cancer; unlike estrogen, they do not significantly increase high-density lipoprotein cholesterol levels, but like estrogen, they reduce total and low-density lipoprotein cholesterol levels
Calcitonin	Increases bone density in the spine, distal radius, and femoral neck	Decreases risk of vertebral and nonvertebral fractures by approximately 30%	Limited data from randomized trials; approved for treatment but not prevention of osteoporosis; efficacy may wane with long-term use
Calcium and vitamin D supplementation and exercise	Generally preserves or increases bone density at various sites	May decrease fracture rates, but data from clinical trials are limited	Necessary for maintaining bone and preventing accelerated bone loss; diverse additional health benefits

Reproduced by permission from Manson JE, Martin KA. Clinical practice. Postmenopausal hormone-replacement therapy. *N Engl J Med* 2001;345:34.

    4. *Lifestyle changes: Astronauts in microgravity lose 1% of bone mass per month; it is felt, therefore, that weight-bearing exercise is beneficial in preventing osteoporosis.*[9]

III.   Known Risks of Hormone Replacement Therapy

A. Venous thromboembolism (VTE)

    1. *Etiology is uncertain but is felt to be associated with estrogen-induced hypercoagulable states.*[9,10]

    2. *Observational studies indicate an increased risk of 2 to 3.5-fold for VTE with HRT.*[10]

    3. *The HERS study showed a risk of 2.7 for VTE among women in the estrogen/progesterone arm of the study.*[3]

    4. *VTE was increased fivefold in the first 90 days following myocardial infarction. Clinicians should suspend use of HRT or provide VTE prophylaxis during hospitalization for an acute coronary event.*[1,10]

    5. *Idiopathic VTE is not common in women over age 50; however, the absolute risk associated with HRT is low.*

B. Endometrial cancer

    1. *Its etiology is consistent with the estrogen receptors present in endometrial tissue resulting in a thickened endometrium and the possible development of atypical endometrial hyperplasia, considered a premalignant condition, in the presence of circulating estrogen.*

    2. *Observational studies find an increased risk of eightfold to tenfold in long-term users (greater than ten years) of unopposed estrogen therapy, (46 per 10,000 women).*[1]

    3. *The PEPI study showed that 24% of the women in the unopposed estrogen arm of the study developed atypical endometrial hyperplasia versus only 1% in the placebo arm of the study.*[1,2]

    4. *The addition of a progestin, which opposes the effect of estrogen on the endometrium, eliminates the associated increased risk and is considered necessary for women with an intact uterus.*[9] *(See IV.A.4. Probable Risks—Breast Cancer.)*

C. Breast cancer

    1. *Estrogen receptors and progesterone receptors in the breast make it sensitive to circulating HRT.*

    2. *A meta-analysis of 51 international case control and cohort studies found no appreciable increased risk of breast cancer in women on short-term estrogen replacement therapy (less than five years).*[1]

    3. *Long-term use of estrogen replacement therapy (greater than five years) did show an increased risk of 35%.*[1]

    4. *Recent data from the ongoing WHI study suggests an increased risk of 26% in women on combination hormone replacement therapy.*[6]

    5. *Given a decreased risk of endometrial cancer but a probable increase in the risk of breast cancer, guidelines regarding HRT in women with an intact uterus are expected to be*

forthcoming from the American College of Obstetricians and Gynecologists.

6. *SERMs may be an alternative to HRT for women at risk for breast cancer.*[8]

IV. Probable Risks Associated with Hormone Replacement Therapy

A. Gallbladder disease

1. *In observational studies, the risk of gallstones or cholecystectomy is increased by a factor of 2 to 3 in women on ERT.*[1]

2. *The HERS study found a 38% increased risk of gallbladder disease in women on combination estrogen/progestin.*[3]

V. Risks and Benefits Requiring Further Evidence

A. Cardiovascular disease: Randomized trials of HRT have not been able to confirm the cardiovascular benefits (35 to 50% lower risks) previously reported by three decades of observational studies.[1,10]

1. *Randomized trials reported physiological changes of estrogen.*

   a. Estrogen receptors in cardiovascular tissue may protect against atherosclerosis and ischemic diseases through regulation of vasomotor tone and response to injury.[10]

   b. In the liver, receptors act to reduce plasma levels of low density lipoprotein (LDL) by 10 to 14% and increase plasma levels of high density lipoprotein (HDL) by 7 to 8%.[10]

   c. The increase in HDL is attenuated with the addition of medroxyprogesterone (MPA) to estrogen; this attenuation is not realized with natural progesterone.[10]

   d. Favorable effects of estrogen include reduced levels of Lp(a) lipoprotein, inhibited oxidation of LDL, improved endothelial vascular function, and decreased postmenopausal fibrinogen.[1,9,10]

   e. Negative effects on cardiovascular biomarkers include increased triglyceride levels by 20%, activated coagulation through increased factor VII, prothrombin, and fibrinopeptide, and increased levels of C-reactive protein (a marker associated with increased risk of cardiovascular events).[10]

   f. Evidence is insufficient to determine whether differences in preparations, dosages, mode of administration, or type of progestins impact clinical CVD endpoints.[10]

2. *Secondary prevention: Information is based on the large randomized Heart and Estrogen/Progestin Replacement Study (HERS).*[3] *This is the first secondary prevention trial designed to evaluate the effect of combined estrogen and progestin HRT on the risk of clinical cardiovascular events, the overall rate of death from coronary causes, and nonfatal myocardial infarction in 2,763 women with documented coronary heart disease (CHD).*

   a. No reduction in risk of cardiovascular events was seen with HRT in women with preexisting CHD.

   b. Subgroups with elevated baseline serum Lp(a) lipoprotein levels may benefit from HRT, but additional evidence is needed.

    c. Subgroups with preexisting hypertension and prothrombin mutation may be at significantly higher risk for cardiovascular events, but additional evidence is needed.

    d. In the HERS study, a 50% increase in the risk of CHD events was noted in the HRT group in the first year of therapy. This was followed by an unexplained decreased risk, possibly due to accelerated events in susceptible women leaving a lower risk group for follow-up.[1,3,10]

    e. The Papworth Hormone Replacement Therapy Atherosclerosis Study[5] confirms a slight increase in cardiovascular events in the HRT group and no benefit in either the HRT or placebo group.

    f. The Estrogen Replacement and Atherosclerosis (ERA) trial found no effect on the progression of CHD in either the estrogen alone, combination HRT, or placebo groups.[4,10]

3. *Primary prevention: Large-scale randomized studies (e.g., the Women's Health Initiative (WHI)[6] study and the Postmenopausal Estrogen/Progestin Interventions (PEPI)[2] study evaluated cardiovascular events in postmenopausal women without preexisting coronary heart disease.*

    a. Interim analysis found a slight increase in myocardial infarctions, strokes, and vascular thromboembolic events in the HRT group.[1,10]

    b. Additional short-term trials found an insignificant increase of cardiovascular events in HRT groups.[10]

    c. Additional evidence is necessary for definitive practice guidelines.

4. *Preventive strategies for CHD for postmenopausal women with and without preexisting disease.*[10]

    a. Recommendations from the American Heart Association and the American College of Cardiology[10]

       i. All women: Lifestyle approaches include smoking avoidance, proper nutrition, and regular exercise.

       ii. Women who do not meet target lipid or blood pressure levels with lifestyle interventions should add pharmacotherapy, that is, lipid-lowering agents and antihypertensives.

       iii. Women with CHD should consider therapies to include antiplatelet agents, anticoagulants (when indicated), beta-blockers, and ACE inhibitors.

       iv. Education and preventive therapies should be a part of clinical practice for all menopausal women. American Heart Association studies found 90% of participants wanted to discuss cardiovascular disease (CVD) and prevention with their physician, but only 30% did.

    b. Secondary prevention strategies

       i. HRT should not be initiated for secondary prevention of CVD.

       ii. Established noncoronary risks and benefits and patient preference should guide decisions to continue or stop long-term HRT in women with CVD.

       iii. Discontinuance of HRT or VTE prophylaxis should be considered in women who develop an acute CVD event or are immobilized while on HRT. Resumption of HRT should be based on established noncoronary risks and benefits and patient preference.

    c. Primary prevention strategies

        i. Definitive evidence from randomized clinical trials is necessary for primary prevention recommendations.

        ii. Insufficient data exist to suggest that HRT should be initiated for the sole purpose of primary prevention of CVD.

        iii. Initiation and continuation of HRT should be based on established noncoronary risks and benefits, possible coronary risks and benefits, and patient preference.

B. Colorectal cancer.

    1. *Observational studies suggest a reduction of 8 to 33% in the risk of colorectal cancer with the use of HRT.*[1]

    2. *Definitive data are insufficient to provide evidence-based recommendations.*

C. Cognitive degeneration.

    1. *Recent observational studies failed to support previous findings suggesting a positive effect on cognitive dysfunction and Alzheimer's disease in women on HRT.*[1]

    2. *A recent randomized trial found no benefit of HRT in the treatment of mild to moderate Alzheimer's disease.*[1]

    3. *Definitive evidence is forthcoming from the Women's Health Initiative study evaluating the effect of HRT on memory loss and cognitive decline.*[6]

D. Type II diabetes mellitus.

    1. *Observational studies suggest a risk reduction in Type II diabetes mellitus with the use of HRT.*[1]

    2. *Evidence from randomized clinical trials is necessary before making practice recommendations.*

E. Ovarian cancer.

    1. *Limited observational studies suggest an increased risk of ovarian cancer with HRT.*[1]

    2. *Definitive data from randomized studies are required before making clinical practice recommendations.*

VI. **Hormone Therapies**

A. Estrogen verses estrogen/progestin combination therapies

    1. *Estrogen therapies*

        a. Estrogen therapy is appropriate for women following a hysterectomy.

        b. Therapies are a pharmacologic substitution of an estrogen analogue for the missing physiologic estradiol—not replacement of estradiol itself.[9]

        c. Available estrogen analogues include conjugated estrogens, estrogen substitutes (diethylstilbestrol), synthetic estrogens (ethinyl estradiol or derivatives), and micronized estradiol.

        d. Regimens associated with low risk of complications are those with the lowest effective dose in cyclic (25 days per month) or continuous daily dosing.[9]

        e. The lowest dose recommended for osteoporosis prevention is 0.625 mg conjugated estrogen orally, 0.01 mg or 0.02 mg ethinyl estradiol orally per day, or transdermal patches

0.05 mg once or twice per week. A clinical trial evaluating the effectiveness of half the preceding dose on osteoporosis prevention is ongoing.[1]

 f. Increase the dose slowly as needed to control quality of life.

 g. Vaginal inserts can specifically address vaginal atrophy.

  i. Premarin vaginal cream 0.625 mg/gm, 1/2 applicator twice per week for 8 to 12 weeks; repeat as indicated. The amount of uptake into circulating systemic estrogen is undetermined.

  ii. Estring TM vaginal insert is a polyurethane ring providing continuous delivery of micronized estrodial. Dose is 0.25 micrograms per day to the vaginal mucosa. Minimal systemic uptake is seen after the first 24 hours. The ring is replaced every 90 days. Estring is recommended for urogenital symptom control.[8]

  iii. Vagifem is a vaginal tablet with 75 micrograms of estrodial per tablet. Dosing is 1 tablet inserted vaginally daily for 1 week, decreasing to 1 tablet twice weekly as maintenance dose. Vagifem may be used as an alternative to Estring for control of urogenital symptoms.[8]

 2. *Combination estrogen/progestin therapies*

  a. Combination therapy is appropriate for women with an intact uterus.

  b. Progestin is available as medroxyprogesterone acetate (MPA) (Provera), micronized progesterone synthesized from a plant source (Prometrium), or as norethindrone acetate in a combination transdermal patch (CombiPatch).

  c. Regimens associated with low risk of complications while maintaining osteoporosis and endometrial cancer prevention are cyclic dosing of 15 days of estrogen alone followed by 10 days of combination estrogen and progesterone per month or continuous low dose combination estrogen and progesterone daily.[9]

  d. Cyclic dosing with estrogen is prescribed as:

   i. MPA 5 mg or 10 mg orally day 16 through 25

   ii. Prometrium® 100 mg or 200 mg orally day 16 through 25.

  e. Continuous dosing with estrogen is prescribed as:

   i. MPA 2.5 mg or 5 mg orally, daily

   ii. Prometrium® 100 mg or 200 mg orally, daily

   ii. Norethindrone acetate 0.14 mg or 0.25 mg transdermally, daily.

B. Natural hormones

 1. *Specifically compounded naturally prepared estrogens prepared according to prescription.*

 2. *Definitive randomized clinical trials are needed to determine the efficacy and safety of natural estrogens.*

VII. **Prescriptive Hormone Alternatives**

A. Selective Estrogen Receptor Modulators (SERMs)

 1. *Tamoxifen (Nolvadex®)*

  a. Breast chemoprevention therapy is an alternative to HRT for menopausal women at increased risk for breast cancer. (See Chapter 10, Counseling about risk management.)

  b. Tamoxifen is proven to decrease breast cancer risk.

    c. Tamoxifen may increase menopausal symptoms.

    d. Tamoxifen is comparable to estrogen in reducing bone fractures.

2. *Raloxifene (Evista®)*

    a. Definitive evidence found raloxifene to be comparable to estrogen in reducing bone fractures.[1]

    b. An ongoing randomized study is evaluating raloxifene and tamoxifen for breast cancer prevention in postmenopausal women at risk for the disease.[8]

    c. The safety of long-term use and breast cancer risks is unknown.

    d. Definitive evidence of the safety of raloxifene in women with a personal history of breast cancer is not available.

    e. Dose: 60 mg orally, daily.

B. Bisphosphonates

1. *Alendronate (Fosamax®) as the sodium salt*

    a. It is indicated in the prevention and treatment of osteoporosis.

    b. Patient education is necessary to prevent side effects due to inappropriate administration.

    c. It is now available as a weekly dose to decrease side effects.

    d. Dose:

       i. 70 mg orally, weekly—prevention and treatment

       ii. 5 mg orally, daily—prevention

       iii. 10 mg orally, daily—treatment

2. *Risedronate (Actonel®) as the sodium salt*

    a. It is indicated for the prevention and treatment of osteoporosis.

    b. Patient education is necessary to prevent side effects due to inappropriate administration.

    c. Dose: 5 mg/day orally.

C. Antidepressant therapy

1. *Venlafaxine extended release (Effexor XR®)*

    a. Decreases the intensity and frequency of the majority of classic menopausal symptoms[8]

    b. Does not affect urogenital menopausal symptoms

    c. Usual dosage: 37.5 mg orally, daily—may increase to 75 mg daily after one to two weeks if necessary

2. *Paroxetine extended release (Paxil CR®)*

    a. Alternative to Effexor XR for nonhormonal control of classic menopausal symptoms

    b. Does not affect urogenital symptoms

    c. Associated with greater weight gain than Effexor XR, therefore, may be indicated in women with decreased appetite

    d. Dose: 10 mg to 20 mg orally, daily

D. Others

1. *Clonidine (Catapres T®)*

    a. Assists in control of vasodilation symptoms.

    b. Precautions: is an antihypertensive and should not be used in patients with low blood pressure. Safe in normotensive patients.

    c. Dose: 0.1 to 0.4 mg/day orally in divided doses BID/TID.

    d. Dose: 0.1 to 0.3 mg/day transdermal patch.

FIGURE 8.1 Algorithm for Identifying Appropriate Candidates for Short-Term and Long-Term Use of Postmenopausal Hormone Replacement Therapy (HRT)

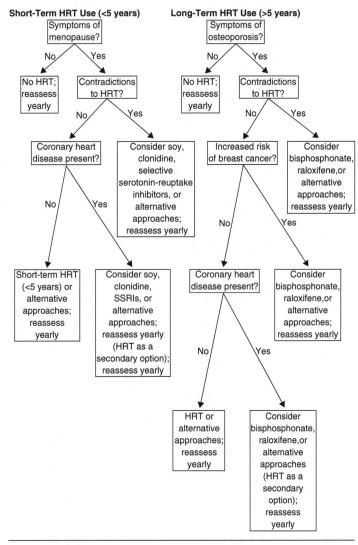

Reproduced by permission from Manson JE, Martin KA, Clinical practice. Postmenopausal hormone-replacement therapy. *N Engl J Med* 2001;345:37.

    2. *Bellamine S*

        a. 40 mg phenobarbital/0.2 mg belladonna/0.6 mg ergotamine per tablet.

        b. Assists in control of vasodilation symptoms, mood disturbances, and sleep disruption.

        c. Precautions: can be habit-forming and can cause sleepiness. Monitor for depression.

        d. Dose: 1 tablet orally one to two times daily. Begin with evening dose and add morning dose as necessary.

VIII. Practice Guidelines (Algorithm)

A. Summary recommendations.

1. *Clinicians should initiate discussion regarding health promotion, age-related chronic disease prevention, and menopause with all perimenopausal and postmenopausal patients.*

2. *Prevention and treatment options should be based on health status, personal and family history and risk factors, and patient preference.*

3. *Lifestyle changes must be an integral part of the health plan including smoking avoidance, nutritional guidance, stress reduction, and exercise.*

4. *An awareness of patient involvement with complementary and alternative therapies is necessary, and an integrated approach is recommended.*

B. Algorithm guides HRT recommendations: Definitive evidence regarding the efficacy and safety of HRT in disease prevention and health promotion is ongoing. An example of such is seen in Figure 8.1.

References

1. Manson J, Martin K. Postmenopausal hormone-replacement therapy. *N Engl J Med* 2001;345:34–40.

2. The Postmenopausal Estrogen/Progestin Interventions (PEPI) Trial. The Writing Group for the PEPI Trial. Effects of estrogen or estrogen/progestin regimens on heart disease risk factors in postmenopausal women. *JAMA* 1995;273:199–208.

3. Heart and Estrogen/Progestin Replacement Study (HERS) Research Group. Randomized trial of estrogen and progestin for secondary prevention of coronary heart disease in postmenopausal women. *JAMA* 1998;280:605–613.

4. Estrogen Replacement and Atherosclerosis (ERA) Trial Research Group. Effects of estrogen replacement on the progression of coronary artery atherosclerosis. *N Engl J Med* 2000;343:522–529.

5. Papworth Hormone-Replacement Therapy Atherosclerosis Study. Research Group. Transdermal estradiol alone or with norethindrone hormone replacement therapy for secondary prevention of coronary artery disease in postmenopausal women. *Eur Heart J* 2000;21(suppl):212.

6. Writing Group for the Women's Health Initiative Investigators. Risks and benfits of estrogen plus progestin in healthy postmenopausal women. Principal results from the Women's Health Initiative randomized controlled trial. *JAMA* 2002;288:321–333.

7. Women's International Study of Long Duration Oestrogen after Menopause. Available at: *www.nih.gov/wisldom/.htn.*

8. National Surgical Adjuvant Breast and Bowel Project. The study of Tamoxifen and Raloxifene (STAR). Available at: *www.nsabp.pitt.edu.*

9. Isselbacher K, Braunwald E, et al. *Harrison's Principals of Internal Medicine.* 13th ed. New York: McGraw-Hill, Inc:2001;2033–2034.

10. Mosca L, Collins P, et al. Hormone replacement therapy and cardiovascular disease: A statement for healthcare professionals from the American Heart Association. *Circulation* 2001;104:499.

Prophylactic Mastectomy

Sue Ely, RN
Magee-Womens Hospital
University of Pittsburgh Medical Center Health System
Pittsburgh, PA

I. Prophylactic mastectomy as a prevention method for breast cancer is controversial and not well studied. With the advent of genetic testing for breast cancer, we are now better able to identify the population of women who may benefit from this prevention modality.

II. **Indications for Prophylactic Mastectomy.**
   A. Historic indications for prophylactic mastectomy include:
      1. *Breast pain*
      2. *Mammographically "Dense" breasts*
      3. *Multiple breast biopsies regardless of histopathology*
      4. *A host of other factors, many not associated with an increased risk of breast cancer*
   B. Today many insurance plans will not pay for this procedure unless the indication is clearly identified.

III. **Elimination of the Risk of Breast Cancer.**
   A. Identifying who is at high risk

Previously this was a challenge with no consistent definition of high risk.[1] Many women overestimate their risk using factors such as age, parity, and family history.[2] The discovery of the BRCA1 and BRCA2 genes have helped to quantify further this high-risk group. (Other chapters in this book review indepth the factors that increase risk.)

   B. BRCA1/2 mutation carriers
      1. *Average lifetime risk for all women is approximately 12%.[3]*
      2. BRCA1 and BRCA2 mutation carriers, average lifetime risk is between 40 and 80%.[4]
      3. *In women whose family histories suggest an autosomal dominant pattern, 85% are found to carry BRCA1 or BRCA2 mutations with 15% of these patients possibly carrying an unidentified genetic mutation.*
   C. Previous diagnosis of breast cancer
      1. *The stage of breast cancer, multifocality, presence of ductal carcinoma in situ, atypical ductal epithelial hyperplasia in the remaining breast, and family history may influence a decision for prophylactic mastectomy.[5]*
      2. *It is controversial whether prophylactic surgery of the contralateral breast should be done in node-positive breast cancer and in patients with metastatic disease because of their predictable short survival.*
   D. Proliferate benign disease
      1. *This includes hyperplasia with or without atypia.[6]*
      2. *It does not include a history of lobular carcinoma in situ or ductal carcinoma in situ.*

TABLE 9.1	Indications for Prophylactic Mastectomy	
	Strong Indicators	**Relative Indicators**
History of invasive breast cancer	• Biopsy showing DCIS, LCIS, or ADH in remaining breast • One or more first-degree relatives with breast cancer • Combination of above	• Large pendulous remaining breast (causing shoulder and/or back pain) • Multiple breast biopsies causing difficulty with screening • Desires bilateral reconstruction
No history of invasive breast cancer	• Bilateral, multi-focal DCIS • Unilateral DCIS or LCIS with contralateral ADH • Bilateral ADH and first-degree relative with premenopausal breast cancer • Any of the above with BRCA1 or BRCA2 mutation	• Bilateral ADH in premenopausal women • No family history of breast cancer • Nonproliferative histology, but two or more first-degree relatives with breast cancer

Shestak K, Medalie D, Williams S. Prophylactic mastectomy. In: Vogel VG, ed. *Management of Patients at High Risk for Breast Cancer.* Malden, MA: Blackwell Science Inc; 2001;183–200.

IV. **Indications for Prophylactic Mastectomy: Women with a History of Breast Cancer and Women without a History of Breast Cancer (Table 9.1).**

    A. Each category identifies both strong and relative indications for prophylactic mastectomy.

    B. It is very rare for a woman's calculated lifetime risk of breast cancer to ever exceed 25 to 30% in the absence of a genetic mutation.

V. **Management Options for the High-Risk Woman.**

    A. Prophylactic surgery.

        1. *Until recently no prospective studies had been done on the effectiveness of prophylactic mastectomy.*

        2. *Hartmann et al reported a study of women at high risk who underwent bilateral prophylactic mastectomy.*[7]

            a. This cohort study included all women with a family history of breast cancer who underwent bilateral prophylactic mastectomy at the Mayo Clinic between 1960 and 1993.

            b. Women were divided into two groups—high risk and moderate risk—on the basis of family history.

    c. A control study of the sisters of the high-risk probands and the Gail model were used to predict the number of breast cancers expected in these two groups in the absence of prophylactic mastectomy.

    d. The study identified 639 women with a family history of breast cancer who had undergone bilateral prophylactic mastectomy: 214 at high risk and 425 at moderate risk.

    e. The median length of follow-up was 14 years.

    f. The median age at prophylactic mastectomy was 42 years.

    g. According to the Gail model, 37.4 breast cancers were expected in the moderate-risk group; 4 breast cancers occurred (reduction in risk, 89.5 percent; P<0.001).

    h. Investigators compared the number of breast cancers among the 214 high-risk probands with the number among their 403 sisters who had not undergone prophylactic mastectomy.

        i. Of these sisters, 38.7 percent (156) had been given a diagnosis of breast cancer (115 cases were diagnosed before the respective proband's prophylactic mastectomy, 38 were diagnosed afterward, and the time of the diagnosis was unknown in 3 cases).

        ii. By contrast, breast cancer was diagnosed in 1.4 percent (3 of 214) of the probands.

        iii. Thus, prophylactic mastectomy was associated with a reduction in the incidence of breast cancer of at least 90 percent.

    i. In women with a high risk of breast cancer on the basis of family history, prophylactic mastectomy can significantly reduce the incidence of breast cancer.

B. The only prospective study[8] looked at women with BRCA1 or BRCA2 mutations.

    1. Women with a pathogenic BRCA1 or BRCA2 mutations were enrolled in a breast cancer surveillance program at the Rotterdam Family Cancer Clinic.

    2. At the time of enrollment, none of the women had a history of breast cancer.

    3. Seventy-six of these women eventually underwent prophylactic mastectomy, and the other 63 remained under regular surveillance.

    4. The effect of mastectomy on the incidence of breast cancer was analyzed by the Cox proportional-hazards method in which mastectomy was modeled as a time-dependent covariate.

    5. No cases of breast cancer were observed following prophylactic mastectomy after a mean follow-up of 2.9 ± 1.4 years.

    6. Eight breast cancers developed in women under regular surveillance after a mean follow-up of 3.0 ± 1.5 years (P=0.003; hazard ratio, 0; 95 percent confidence interval, 0 to 0.36).

    7. The actuarial mean five-year incidence of breast cancer among all women in the surveillance group was 17 ± 7 percent.

    8. On the basis of an exponential model, the yearly incidence of breast cancer in this group was 2.5 percent.

9. *The observed number of breast cancers in the surveillance group was consistent with the expected number (ratio of observed to expected cases, 1.2; 95 percent confidence interval, 0.4 to 3.7; P=0.80).*

10. *In women with a BRCA1 or BRCA2 mutation, prophylactic bilateral total mastectomy reduces the incidence of breast cancer at three years of follow-up.*

C. In retrospective studies, there is also a reduction in breast cancer risk in women who carry BRCA1 mutations and who undergo bilateral oophorectomy;[9] the probable cause is a decrease in hormone exposure.

D. Removal of occult cancers: After prophylactic mastectomy, 5% of specimens detect occult breast cancer.[5]

E. Cancerphobia or a high level of anxiety or distress over the risk of developing breast cancer may be an appropriate indication.[2]

1. *This should be used in conjunction with other high risk criteria.*

2. *For some patients the lifelong fear of surveillance for breast cancer outweighs the cost and risk of prophylactic mastectomy.*

3. *Prophylactic mastectomy should only be performed when appropriate psychological counseling has been obtained.*

F. Multiple breast biopsies.

VI. **What to Consider When Counseling a Woman Regarding Prophylactic Mastectomy.**

A. Quantify risk in terms of the probability that a woman will develop breast cancer in her lifetime using either an empiric or an analytic estimate.[10]

B. Provide the woman and her family with accurate information (using a multidisciplinary approach with surgical consults as well as medical genetics and social service) regarding her risk and methods to decrease that risk such as intensive surveillance, chemoprevention, and prophylactic mastectomy.

C. Remember to provide this information in a way to heighten awareness instead of increasing anxiety.[2]

D. Discuss the risks and benefits of prophylactic mastectomy.[11]

E. Be attentive to the psychological needs of the woman and her family and provide counseling when appropriate.

VII. **Surgical Approaches.**

A. Definition of prophylactic mastectomy: Surgical removal of the breast when no cancer is present with the goal of prevention of breast cancer or reducing the risk of breast cancer.[4]

B. Operative techniques.

1. *Subcutaneous mastectomy*

a. This procedure includes removal of all breast tissue including the tail of Spence and the nipple areolar complex.[4, 5]

b. On average, 10% or more of the breast tissue remains.

2. *Total/simple mastectomy*
   a. This procedure includes removal of breast gland, nipple/areolar complex.
   b. Ninety-five percent of the breast tissue is removed.[4]
   c. With greatly improved nipple reconstruction techniques, total mastectomy is becoming the treatment of choice.
   d. Skin-sparing mastectomy is a modification of total mastectomy in which only skin at risk of harboring glandular breast tissue is excised.[4]

3. *Reconstruction options*
   a. A transverse rectus abdominus musculocutaneous (TRAM) flap is the most common autologous reconstruction.[5]
      i. This procedure involves use of the rectus abdominus muscle to create a new breast mound.
      ii. This reconstruction can be tunneled through the abdominal area to the breast region or transferred as a free flap.
      iii. This procedure has the most natural cosmetic outcome.
      iv. Patients note tightness and/or pain in the abdomen, but this resolves with time.
   b. Tissue expander/implants.
      i. Creating a breast with a saline-filled implant usually requires tissue expansion prior to placement of the implant and is a two-step procedure.
      ii. Implant complications most frequently seen are contractures or firmness of the reconstructed breast and asymmetry or rupture.

VIII. **Risks of Prophylactic Mastectomy.**
   A. Physical
      1. *Poor cosmesis: flap necrosis, asymmetry, and capsular contracture*[4, 5]
      2. *Hematomas, seromas, skin numbness, and infection*[4]
      3. *Reoperations—appears to be less common in reconstruction after total mastectomy versus subcutaneous mastectomy*
   B. Psychosocial complications
      1. *Mastectomy is a mutilating procedure, and many studies report that women express feelings of depression, anger, and loss in addition to sexual dysfunction.*
      2. *With the advance in reconstructive techniques, many of the preceding feelings are minimized.*
      3. *It is important to evaluate each woman individually and allow her enough time to make this decision and explore options for reconstruction.*
      4. *Unfortunately, the cost of reconstructive surgery is quite high, and insurance companies need to be shown objective evidence to justify the cost. All patients need to explore their individual policies for coverage.*

IX. **Benefits of Surgery.**
   A. Hartmann et al reported in their Mayo clinic study[7] that 609 women completed a quality of life questionnaire.

1. *Seventy percent of all women who underwent prophylactic mastectomy were satisfied or very satisfied with their decision for prophylactic surgery.*
2. *Most reported a significant decrease in their anxiety and worry over possible breast cancer development.*

X. Summary.

A. The decision to undergo prophylactic mastectomy is difficult for both the patient and her physician who is counseling her.

B. The decision needs to be based on a woman's objective risk profile and factors such as personal values, anxiety over eventual cancer development, and desire for reconstruction.

C. This requires both education and counseling from a multidisciplinary group and allowing the woman sufficient time to make an informed decision.

D. In much recent literature, the population best suited for prophylactic mastectomy are women at high risk for the eventual development of cancer.

References

1. Houshmand SL, Campbell CT, Briggs SE, McFadden AWJ, Al-Tweigeri T. Prophylactic Mastectomy and Genetic Testing: An Update. *Oncology Nursing Forum* 2000;27(10):1537–49.

2. Vogel VG. Counseling the high-risk woman. In: Stoll BA, ed. *Reducing Breast Cancer Risk in Women.* Dordrecht, The Netherlands: Kluwer Academic Publishers; 1995;69–80.

3. Vogel VG, Yeomans AC. Clinical Management of women at increased risk of breast cancer. *Breast Cancer Res Treat* 1993;28:195–210.

4. Blanchard DK, Hartmann LC. Prophylactic mastectomy for women at high risk for breast cancer, *Breast Diseases: A Year Book Quarterly* 2001;11:361–362.

5. Shestak KC, Medalie DA, Williams SL. Prophylactic mastectomy. In: Vogel VG, ed. *Management of Patients at High Risk for Breast Cancer.* Malden, MA: Blackwell Science Inc; 2001;183–200.

6. Swain M. Noninvasive breast cancer: Part 2. Lobular carcinoma in situ-incidence, presentation, guidelines to treatment. *Oncology* 1989;3:35–40.

7. Hartmann LC, Schaid DJ, Woods JE, et al. Efficacy of bilateral prophylactic mastectomy in women with a family history of breast cancer. *N Engl J Med* 1999;340:77–84.

8. Meijers-Heijboer M, van Geel B, van Putten WLJ, et al. Breast cancer after prophylactic bilateral mastectomy in women with BRCA1 or BRCA2 mutation. *N Engl J Med* 2001;345:159–164.

9. Rebbeck TR, Lynch HT, Neuhausen SL, et al. Prophylactic oophorectomy in carriers of BRCA1 or BRCA2 mutations. *New Engl J Med* 2002;346:1616–1622.

10. O'Neill S. Quantitative breast cancer risk assessment. In: Vogel VG, ed. *Management of Patients at High Risk for Breast Cancer.* Malden, MA: Blackwell Science Inc; 2001;63–93.

11. Iglehart JD. Prophylactic mastectomy. In: Harris J, Lippman M, Morrow M, Osborne CK, eds. *Diseases of the Breast.* Philadelphia, PA: J. B. Lippincott; 2000;255–264.

chapter 10

Counseling about Risk Management

Robin L. Coyne, MS, APRN, BC
Family Nurse Practitioner
Cancer Prevention Center
The University of Texas M. D. Anderson Cancer Center
Houston, TX

Therese Bevers, MD
Medical Director
Cancer Prevention Center
The University of Texas M. D. Anderson Cancer Center
Houston, TX

I.   **Introduction**

As health care approached the new millennium, medical research provided the opportunity to refine the approach to preventing breast cancer. In 1998, the Food and Drug Administration approved the selective estrogen receptor modulator, tamoxifen citrate, for the reduction of breast cancer risk. Women who are at increased risk for breast cancer are now able to reduce their risk with a chemopreventive agent. Subsequently, primary prevention strategies for breast cancer have changed. It is important for the clinician to be aware of these changes and to effectively incorporate new standards into practice. This chapter provides an overview of the risk assessment process and reviews current guidelines for both risk reduction of breast cancer and chemoprevention counseling.

II.   **Risk Assessment Process**

    A.   Breast cancer risk assessment has become the basis from which risk reduction and screening recommendations are made. Risk reduction strategies are based on individual breast cancer risk. Analysis of risk factors and family history allows the healthcare provider to assign individuals to average risk, increased population risk, or increased familial risk subsets.

    B.   It is important to determine the appropriate setting in which risk assessment should be conducted.

        1.   *Breast cancer risk assessments should be performed during the annual breast examination.*

        2.   *The process may also be initiated within the context of periodic health examinations.*

        3.   *Women presenting with breast complaints or abnormalities will benefit from risk assessment because:*

            a.   Knowledge of the patient's risk for breast cancer may help guide the clinician in making management decisions (i.e., a 25-year-old female with a palpable breast mass reporting a mother and sister diagnosed with breast cancer in their thirties will be managed aggressively. Biopsy would likely be more appropriate than short-term observation.).

            b.   The risk assessment process may provide reassurance to patients of average risk who perceive an elevated risk for breast cancer.

    C.   The first step in the risk assessment process is to identify individuals with a strong family history of breast cancer. These women will benefit from information on genetic risk (see Chapter 3).

        1.   *Obtain a detailed family history.*

            a.   Ascertain patterns or trends suggestive of hereditary breast or ovarian cancer syndrome (i.e., maternal versus paternal, unilateral versus bilateral breast cancer, age of diagnosis).

            b.   If a hereditary breast or ovarian cancer syndrome is suspected, refer the patient and her family for genetic risk counseling.

        2.   *The National Comprehensive Cancer Network, a group of experts from 18 leading cancer centers throughout the United*

States, has established guidelines for the evaluation and management of patients with a familial or inherited predisposition to breast cancer. An overview of criteria which are suggestive of hereditary breast or ovarian cancer syndromes, warranting further review, is shown in Table 10.1. Key components of the family history, as specified in section 5 of the table, may be applied easily in a general practice setting by clinicians who are caring for women without a personal history of breast or ovarian cancer.[1]

D. The Gail Risk Assessment Model.

1. The Gail model was developed at the National Cancer Institute.

2. The modified version of the tool was validated during the Breast Cancer Prevention Trial (BCPT) and can be used to identify women who are at increased risk for breast cancer.[2]

3. A computer program of the model is available for distribution to health care providers via the Internet at http://bcra.nci.nih.gov/brc.[3]

4. The program prompts the user to enter risk factors specific to the individual.

    a. Race.
    b. Current age.
    c. Age at menarche.
    d. Age at first live birth.
    e. Number of first-degree relatives with a history of breast cancer.
    f. Number of previous breast biopsies.
    g. A history of atypical hyperplasia will approximately double a woman's risk for breast cancer as calculated by the Gail model (Table 10.2).[4]

5. An individual's estimated five-year and lifetime risks are calculated and compared to women of the same age and race who are at average risk for breast cancer (Figure 10.1).

6. Increased risk is defined as a five-year risk of 1.7% or greater. A five-year risk of 1.7% equates to the risk of an average 60-year-old woman.[1]

7. The majority of women undergoing breast screening examinations and mammography should be evaluated for breast cancer risk using the Gail model. Exceptions include:

    a. Women under the age of 35.
        i. The model is designed to calculate the risk of women ages 35 through 85 years. Risk factors for women ages 20 through 34 years may be entered, and a calculation will be performed. A disclaimer indicates that no woman under the age of 35 was permitted to enroll in BCPT.
        ii. The use of tamoxifen for the reduction of breast cancer risk has not been studied in women under the age of 35.
        iii. Women less than 35 years of age with a strong family history of breast cancer would benefit from genetic risk assessment and counseling.

    b. Women 85 years of age or older.
        i. The model will not calculate breast cancer risk for women older than 85.

TABLE 10.1 Hereditary Breast and/or Ovarian Cancer (HBOC-A)

HBOC Criteria[g,h]

1. Member of known BRCA1/BRCA2 kindred

2. Personal history of breast cancer + one or more of the following:
   a. Diagnosed age ≤ 40 yr, with or without family history
   b. Diagnosed age ≤ 50 yr or bilateral, with > 1 close blood relative with breast cancer or ≥ 1 close blood relative with ovarian cancer
   c. Diagnosed at any age, with ≥ 2 close blood relatives with ovarian cancer at any age, or breast cancer, especially if ≥ 1 woman is diagnosed before age 50 yr or has bilateral disease
   d. Close male blood relative has breast cancer
   e. If of Ashkenazi Jewish descent and diagnosed age ≤ 50 yr, no additional family history required, or at any age if history of breast and/or ovarian cancer in close blood relative

3. Personal history of ovarian cancer + one or more of the following:
   a. ≥ 1 close blood relative with ovarian cancer
   b. ≥ 1 close female blood relative with breast cancer at age ≤ 50 yr or bilateral breast cancer
   c. ≥ 2 close blood relatives with breast cancer
   d. ≥ 1 close male blood relative with breast cancer
   e. If of Ashkenazi Jewish descent, no additional family history is required

4. Personal history of male breast cancer + one or more of the following:
   a. ≥ 1 close male blood relative with breast cancer
   b. ≥ 1 close female blood relative with breast or ovarian cancer
   c. If of Ashkenazi Jewish descent, no additional family history is required

5. Family history only—one or more of the following:
   a. ≥1 close blood relative with breast cancer age ≤ 40 yr or bilateral breast cancer
   b. ≥ 2 close blood relatives with ovarian cancer
   c. ≥ 2 close blood relatives with breast cancer especially if ≥ 1 is age ≤ 50 yr
   d. ≥ 1 close blood relative with breast cancer ≥ 1 with ovarian cancer, any age
   e. If of Ashkenazi Jewish descent, 1 close relative with breast or ovarian cancer

[g]Criteria suggestive of hereditary breast/ovarian cancer syndrom that warrant further professional evaluation.

[h]When investigating family histories for HBOC, all close relatives on the same side of the family should be included. Close relatives include first-, second-, and third-degree relatives.

Note: All reccomendations are category 2A unless otherwise indicated.

Clinical Trials: NCCN believes that the best management of any cancer patient is in a clinical trial. Participation in clinical trials is especially encouraged.

NCCN Genetics/Familial High-Risk Cancer Screening Guideline, "The Complete Library of NCCN Oncology Practice Guidelines" [CD-ROM]. (2001). Rockledge, Pennsylvania. To view the most recent version of the guideline, go online to www.nccn.org

"These guidelines are a work in progress that will be refined as often as new significant data becomes available."

"The NCCN guidelines are a statement of consensus of its authors regarding their views of currently accepted approaches to treatment. Any clinician seeking to apply or consult any NCCN guideline is expected to use independent medical judgment in the context of individual clinical circumstances to determine any patient's care or treatment. The National Comprehensive Cancer Network makes no warranties of any kind whatsoever regarding their content, use or application and disclaims any responsibility for their application or use in any way."

TABLE 10.2	Breast Lesions and Relative Risk for Invasive Breast Cancer		
No Increased Risk	**Slightly Increased Risk (1.5–2.0×)**	**Moderately Increased Risk (5×)**	**Markedly Increased Risk (10×)**
Adenosis	Hyperplasia (Moderate or florid, solid or papillary)	Atypical hyperplasia (ductal or lobular)	Lobular carcinoma *in situ*
Apocrine metaplasia	Papillomatosis		Atypical hyperplasia with family history of breast cancer
Cysts			
Duct ectasia			
Fibroadenoma			
Fibrosis			
Hyperplasia, mild			
Mastitis			
Squamous metaplasia			

Hunt KK, Robb GL, Strom EA, et al, eds. *M.D. Anderson Cancer Care Series: Breast Cancer.* New York: Springer Verlag; 2001:20–47. Used with permission.

FIGURE 10.1 Breast Cancer Risk

5-YEAR RISK:

- Patient (age 61) 1.3%
- Woman (age 61)—same race and average risk factors 1.1%

Explanation:

Based on the data provided, your patient's estimated risk for invasive breast cancer over the next 5 years is 1.3% compared to that of 1.1% for a woman who is the same age as your patient with average risk factors over the same 5-year period. This also means that your patient's risk of *not* getting breast cancer over the next 5 years is 98.7%.

Your patient's risk for invasive breast cancer of 1.3% would not have been high enough to qualify for the Breast Cancer Prevention Trial. In this trial, women qualified for entry with a 5-year risk of 1.7% or higher.

LIFETIME RISK:

- Patient (to age 90) 6.8%
- Woman (to age 90)—same race and average risk factors 5.6%

Explanation:

Based on the data provided, your patient's estimated risk for invasive breast cancer over her lifetime is 6.8% compared to that of 5.6% for a woman who is the same age as your patient with average risk factors over her lifetime.

Do not confuse the lifetime risk with the 1.7% cutoff point used by the Breast Cancer Prevention Trial. It is the 5-year risk which should be compared to 1.7% rather than the lifetime risk.

      ii. The risks associated with tamoxifen use likely outweigh any estimated benefit as the lifetime risk of breast cancer diminishes as the woman nears the age of 90 and side effects increase in frequency.

  c. Women with a history of invasive breast cancer, lobular carcinoma in situ (LCIS), or ductal carcinoma in situ (DCIS).

      i. These women are known to be at increased risk for invasive breast cancer.

      ii. The Gail model does not assess the risks associated with either a personal history of breast cancer, LCIS, or DCIS.

  d. Women with American College of Radiology abnormal mammographic findings should undergo further evaluation (see Chapter 5).

      i. A highly suspicious finding on mammography must be thoroughly evaluated with tissue sampling performed to rule out carcinoma.

      ii. If the process proves to be benign on excisional biopsy, the Gail model should be calculated taking the histologic findings into consideration and adding one biopsy to the model.

  e. Women with known or suspected genetic predisposition for breast cancer.

      i. The Gail model only solicits family history involving first-degree relatives with breast cancer.

      ii. The Gail model may underestimate the risk of breast cancer if there is a family history suggestive of a BRCA1 or BRCA2 mutation.

8. *The Gail model may be incorporated into the clinical setting.*

  a. Clinic staff (i.e., registered nurses, licensed vocational nurses, and nursing or medical assistants) may be trained to obtain the information necessary for the risk profile. Staff education is essential to assure accuracy of the risk assessment. Several key components should be considered and reinforced.

      i. Age of parity is equivalent to the first live birth. Pregnancies not resulting in live birth should be excluded.

      ii. First-degree relatives with a history of LCIS or DCIS should be counted as a breast cancer diagnosis and entered into the risk assessment profile.

      iii. Fathers or brothers diagnosed with breast cancer should not be included in the calculation. Individuals with a family history of male breast cancer should be referred for genetic counseling.

      iv. Provide guidance on documentation of biopsies. This process is threefold:

        • Should the biopsy be counted? A fine-needle aspiration (FNA) is appropriate to include in the risk profile if it was used for diagnostic evaluation. If the specimen was discarded, it is not counted as a biopsy.

        • A core needle biopsy followed by excisional biopsy is counted as one biopsy, as both were used in the diagnostic evaluation of the same process.

        • The cytology/histology of the previous biopsy is also important. Atypical hyperplasia on breast biopsy carries more risk for breast cancer than benign findings. Hyperplasia alone does not increase risk significantly and should not be counted as atypical hyperplasia.

FIGURE 10.2	Patient Questionnaire: Breast Cancer Risk Assessment

Please answer the following questions prior to your appointment with your healthcare provider. By using this questionnaire, we will estimate your risk for breast cancer. The result of the breast cancer risk assessment will be reviewed with you during your visit. Please circle the appropriate answers.

1. Do you have a personal history of lobular carcinoma-in-situ, ductal carcinoma-in-situ or invasive breast cancer?

   Yes
   No

2. What is your current age?

   _____

3. What was your age at your first menstrual period?

   Unknown
   7 to 11
   12–13
   >13

4. What was your age at your first live birth of a child?

   Unknown
   No births
   < 20
   20–24
   25–30
   > 30

5. How many first-degree relatives do you have with breast cancer? (mother, sister and/or daughter)

   Unknown
   Zero
   1
   > 1

6. Have you ever had a breast biopsy?

   Yes
   No

   How many previous breast biopsies?

   Unknown
   Zero
   1
   > 1

   Have you had at least one biopsy with atypical hyperplasia?

   Unknown
   Yes
   No

7. Please select your race/ethnicity

   White
   Black
   Hispanic
   Asian or
   Pacific
   Islander
   American
   Indian or
   Alaskan native
   Unknown

b. A printed questionnaire (Figure 10.2) that is completed by the patient is also an option to obtain risk factor information.

c. The data are then entered into the computer program by the nursing or ancillary staff, the calculation is made, and the risk assessment is printed.

d. It is the role of the healthcare provider to validate the components of the risk assessment with the patient. This ensures accuracy of the calculation. Accurate documentation is particularly important when determining benign versus atypical biopsy results. Failure to document atypical hyperplasia on previous breast biopsy may result in underestimating the patient's five-year and lifetime risks for breast cancer.

   e. Following an explanation of the risk, the provider may give the patient a copy of the risk assessment. The second copy is signed, dated, and placed in the patient's medical record to serve as medical record documentation.

   f. Ductal lavage may also be used to assess breast cancer risk (see Chapter 6).[5]

III. Risk Assessment Counseling

  A. Thorough risk assessment is crucial to developing an individualized plan for breast cancer risk reduction. Analysis of risk factors and family history allows the healthcare provider to assign patients to average risk, increased risk, or increased familial risk subsets. Risk reduction strategies are based on identifying the individual's breast cancer risk.

  B. Average risk populations.

    1. *The average risk population includes those women with an estimated 5-year risk less than 1.7% per the Gail model and no suspicion of a genetic predisposition.*

    2. *Women at average risk for breast cancer should not be given tamoxifen. There is currently no evidence of benefit in this subset of women. The risks associated with tamoxifen may outweigh any potential benefits.*

    3. *The average woman carries a 12% lifetime risk for breast cancer. This is roughly a one-in-eight chance of developing the disease.[6] As a woman ages, her lifetime risk for breast cancer will gradually diminish as she successfully lives through those years without developing breast cancer.[7]*

    4. *The individual at average risk needs to be reminded of the importance of routine screening. The American Cancer Society recommends annual mammography to begin at the age of 40. A breast examination performed by a trained healthcare provider should either precede or follow the radiologic evaluation.[5]*

    5. *The National Comprehensive Cancer Network's risk-based breast cancer screening guidelines are outlined in Table 10.3.[8]*

    6. *The Gail model risk assessment should be recalculated annually as risk will increase as a woman gets older. Certain risk factor changes (i.e., diagnosis of first-degree relative with breast cancer or recent breast biopsy) may significantly elevate risk.*

  C. Increased familial risk (see Chapters 3 and 11).

    1. *Genetic counseling is recommended for any individual with a family history of cancer suggestive of a Hereditary Breast or Ovarian Cancer Syndrome (BRCA1 or BRCA2).*

    2. *Why should a woman consider genetic risk counseling?*

      a. It provides an individual with a better understanding of her risk for developing not only breast cancer but also ovarian cancer.

      b. Breast cancer risk associated with a genetic mutation is typically significantly greater than the risk calculated by the Gail model. The added knowledge of a genetic predisposition

TABLE 10.3 Breast Cancer Screening and Diagnosis

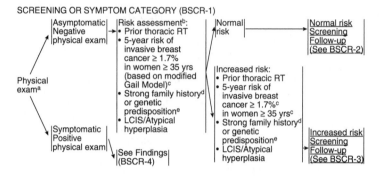

SCREENING OR SYMPTOM CATEGORY (BSCR-1)

SCREENING OR SYMPTOM CATEGORY (BSCR-2)

[a]See Breast Screening Considerations (BSCR-A)

[b]Refer to the NCCN Breast Cancer Risk Reduction Guidelines for a detailed qualitative and quantitative assessment.

[c]Risk Factors Used in the Modified Gail Model (BSCR-B).

[d]For a definition of strong family history, see NCCN Genetics/Cancer Screening Guidelines.

[e]As currently defined in the American Society of Clinical Oncology Guidelines (Statement of the American Society of Clinical Oncology: Genetic testing for cancer susceptibility, adopted on February 20, 1996. J Clin Oncol 14(5):1730–1736, 1996.

Note: All recommendations are category 2A unless otherwise indicated.

Clinical Trials: NCCN believes that the best management of any cancer patient is in a clinical trial. Participation in clinical trials is especially encouraged.

NCCN Breast Cancer Screening Guideline, "The Complete Library of NCCN Oncology Practice Guidelines" [CD-ROM]. (2001). Rockledge, Pennsylvania. To view the most recent version of the guideline, go online to www.nccn.org

"These guidelines are a work in progress that will be refined as often as new significant data becomes available."

"The NCCN guidelines are a statement of consensus of its authors regarding their views of currently accepted approaches to treatment. Any clinician seeking to apply or consult any NCCN guideline is expected to use independent medical judgment in the context of individual clinical circumstances to determine any patient's care or treatment. The National Comprehensive Cancer Network makes no warranties of any kind whatsoever regarding their content, use or application and disclaims any responsibility for their application or use in any way."

      may result in women making significantly different choices in regard to prevention (i.e., prophylactic mastectomy).

  c. In cases of known genetic predisposition, there are risk reduction options in addition to tamoxifen.

Chemoprevention may not be the optimal strategy (i.e., women with known BRCA1 mutations).

3. *Risk reduction strategies for high-risk women include:*
   a. Prophylactic mastectomy.
   b. Prophylactic oophorectomy.
   c. Chemoprevention with tamoxifen was recently identified as effective in women with BRCA2 mutations, reducing the risk by 62%.[9] However, no benefit has been demonstrated for women with BRCA1 mutation. For further information on genetic counseling, refer to Chapter 11.

D. Increased risk.

1. *Increased risk is defined as a personal history of lobular carcinoma in situ or a five-year risk $\geq$ 1.7% using the Gail model.*

2. *Women meeting these criteria should be counseled about their breast cancer risk.*

3. *These same women should also be informed of the option of tamoxifen therapy for breast cancer risk reduction.*

4. *Because a practitioner's contact time with the patient is limited, a brief overview of tamoxifen's risks and benefits can be provided during the breast cancer screening examination. Printed reference material can be given to the patient. The patient should be informed that any hormonal therapy would need to be discontinued before tamoxifen therapy is initiated. For many women, this is the pivotal issue when deciding whether she desires to pursue tamoxifen therapy for risk reduction (see section V, A).*

5. *In general, the patient's options are threefold, although the risks associated with each directive varies. Each option will be reviewed in the context of specific patient risk profiles (see section V, A).*
   a. Continue hormone replacement therapy (if currently on HRT) but provide close clinical follow-up.
   b. Discontinue or avoid initiation of HRT and continue clinical follow-up.
   c. Initiate tamoxifen therapy with continued clinical follow-up.

6. *If the patient indicates an interest in further information and counseling regarding tamoxifen, a "Chemoprevention Consultation" appointment is scheduled at a future date. If the patient is taking HRT, a 3-month drug holiday may be attempted in the interim to assess postmenopausal symptoms that could negatively impact the woman's ability to tolerate tamoxifen.*

IV. **Chemoprevention Counseling**
A. See Chapter 7 for a discussion of the risks and benefits of using tamoxifen for reducing the risk of developing invasive breast cancer.

B. Initial consultation.

1. *Allow sufficient time to conduct the consultation visit.*

2. *The visit takes 45 to 60 minutes as there is a significant amount of information to communicate, and the patient often has numerous questions to be addressed so that she can determine the most appropriate strategy for her.*

3. *Validate the risk factors used in the Gail model risk assessment to both assure accuracy and review the risk assessment with the patient.*

4. *Review past medical history focusing primarily on risk factors associated with the known risks of tamoxifen therapy.*

   a. Uncontrolled diabetes mellitus, hypertension, or atrial fibrillation are associated with increased risk of vascular thrombolic events.

   b. As with HRT, any personal history of a thromboembolic event should be considered a relative contraindication to tamoxifen therapy (i.e., pulmonary embolism, deep vein thrombosis, and cerebral vascular accident).[2]

   c. Undiagnosed uterine bleeding should be evaluated to rule out malignancy, polyps, or another benign process.

5. *Review past surgical and obstetrical/gynecological history.*

   a. Previous hysterectomy nullifies the increased risk for endometrial cancer.

   b. Prior cataract surgery negates the increased risk for cataracts for the eye operated on.

6. *Update current medication list.*

   a. Hormonal therapies (e.g., estrogen, progesterone, combination therapy, or oral contraceptive pills).

      i. The patient will need to discontinue hormonal therapy prior to initiating tamoxifen for risk reduction.

      ii. A three-month washout period is helpful to ascertain if the patient experiences menopausal symptoms.

      iii. If symptoms are persistent, nonhormonal management is initiated, and the effects evaluated. If the patient has significant quality of life issues after discontinuation of the hormones, despite alternatives in management, it is likely that tamoxifen will not be well tolerated.

      iv. Ascertain why the patient is taking a specific hormonal regimen, especially if she is unwilling to stop the medication.

      v. At the time HRT was prescribed, many patients were told it provides protection against myocardial infarction. It is important to educate the patient regarding current data relative to estrogen replacement therapy and cardiovascular disease (see Chapter 8).

   b. Raloxifene (see Chapter 7).

      i. Raloxifene is a selective estrogen receptor modulator drug, which is contraindicated in combination with tamoxifen.

      ii. It is often assumed that raloxifene has the same ability to prevent breast cancer as tamoxifen. Reinforce with the patient the current lack of prospective evidence that raloxifene reduces the risk of breast cancer in high-risk women.[10]

      iii. Current American Society of Clinical Oncology (ASCO) guidelines[11] state that raloxifene should not be used outside of clinical trials for breast cancer risk reduction.

   c. Review similarities and differences among tamoxifen, estrogen replacement therapy, and raloxifene with each woman considering tamoxifen therapy.[2]

      i. Tamoxifen has been proven to reduce the risk of breast cancer while raloxifene's effect is currently being studied, and HRT is likely to increase the risk of the disease if used for more than five years.

      ii. All three hormonal therapies provide some protection from bone loss.

      iii. The risk of thromboembolic events is increased by all three agents.

      iv. The risk for uterine cancer with raloxifene is uncertain while it is well documented that both tamoxifen and unopposed estrogen will increase the risk.

      v. Tamoxifen and raloxifene will not alleviate postmenopausal symptoms and may worsen those symptoms.

      vi. There is insufficient evidence available now to support the ability of HRT, tamoxifen, or raloxifene to reduce the risk of cardiovascular disease.

      vii. Misconceptions about these three treatment regimens may limit a woman's ability to make an informed and knowledgeable decision about taking tamoxifen for breast cancer risk reduction.

7. *Social history.*

   a. Tobacco use will further increase the risk of thromboembolic events.

   b. Heavy alcohol use in combination with tamoxifen therapy may cause hepatic damage, as both are cleared by the liver.

   c. A sedentary lifestyle may result in poor cardiovascular health and increase the risk of blood clots, stroke, and osteoporosis.

8. *Physical examination.*

   a. A comprehensive examination that includes a thorough breast examination is essential prior to initiating therapy.

   b. If an abnormality is identified on clinical breast examination, obtain diagnostic imaging and biopsies as indicated to rule out malignancy.

   c. If clinical breast examination is negative, review and document the results of the most recent mammogram. Schedule patient for a screening mammogram, if one was not performed within the past year.

   d. Perform or refer for gynecologic examination if the woman's uterus is intact.

   e. Evaluate any abnormal uterine bleeding by obtaining an endometrial biopsy and/or transvaginal ultrasound as indicated.

   f. Advise women of childbearing age that tamoxifen should not be initiated if pregnancy is desired. Effective nonhormonal contraception is a necessity to prevent pregnancy while taking tamoxifen.

9. *Develop a plan of care specific to the individual's risks and desires.*

   a. The net effect of tamoxifen therapy is a function of each woman's profile of factors that could lead to adverse events. These include her:

      i. Level of predicted breast cancer risk

      ii. Factors associated with the risk of the other events—age, race, hysterectomy status, and risk for venous thromboembolic events

   b. Women with a high likelihood of a positive net benefit/risk assessment include:[2,12]

      i. Individuals with a personal history LCIS, DCIS, or atypical hyperplasia

       ii. A 5-year breast cancer risk that is greater with increasing age

       iii. Women under the age of 50

       iv. Women over age 49, without a uterus, currently on HRT or a mininal risk for vascular event

    c. *Consideration should be given to personal perspectives.*

       i. Each woman will have her own weighting of the beneficial and detrimental effects.

       ii. Many women at high breast cancer risk are willing to exchange the potential risks of therapy to obtain the potential reduction of breast cancer risk.

V. Management of Women Taking Tamoxifen[13,14]

The role of the healthcare provider is to provide information on breast cancer risk and risk reduction strategies, relating these to the woman's individual risks and concerns. The healthcare provider should attempt to refrain from making the decision. The options should be outlined for the patient, with explanations of the risks and benefits of each, so an informed decision can be made.

    A. Application of risk/benefit profiles to individual clinical situations

---

━━━━━━━━━━ Mary ━━━━━━━━━━

Patient age: 76

Age at first period: 12

Age at first birth: 23

Number of first-degree relatives with breast cancer: None

Number of breast biopsies: 1

Race: White

Estimation of 5-year risk for invasive breast cancer = 1.9%

Estimation of lifetime risk for invasive breast cancer = 3.8%

---

    1. *Mary is a 76-year-old grandmother with an estimated 5-year risk equal to 1.9%. Her lifetime risk equals 3.8%.*

      a. She has an intact uterus and presents annually for well-women examinations.

      b. Mary is currently on HRT for postmenopausal symptoms which have been limited since initiating Prempro® at age 52.

      c. A recent bone density test revealed osteoporosis, and her primary care physician began Fosamax® 70 mg weekly.

      d. As she ages, her 5-year risk and lifetime risk are almost identical.

      e. Mary has three options relative to breast cancer risk reduction.

        i. Discontinue the HRT and give tamoxifen along with the Fosamax®. Although she would reduce her lifetime risk for breast cancer by 49% in relative terms and about 1% in absolute terms, the net benefit would be quite small because the risk of endometrial cancer is approximately 1% with five years of tamoxifen use. There is also increased risk of thrombosis with tamoxifen.

    ii. Discontinue the HRT but continue the Fosamax® for osteoporosis. Long-term HRT use has been associated with increasing risk of breast cancer. Stopping the medication may ultimately help to limit Mary's risk for breast cancer while the Fosamax® is beneficial for her osteoporosis. Any postmenopausal symptoms could be managed with nonhormonal agents.

    iii. Continue both the HRT and Fosamax® as prescribed. Although the long-term hormonal therapy increases the risk of breast cancer by 30 to 40%, many women are hesitant to discontinue the therapy. Given the fact that Mary has survived 76 years without breast cancer, it may be reasonable to continue her present medication regimen although the continued risks of both breast cancer and thrombosis must be considered carefully. Continuation of HRT will provide added protection against osteoporosis and eliminate any postmenopausal symptoms that may have developed on tamoxifen.

Julie

Patient's age: 56

Age at first period: 9

Age at first birth: 26

Number of first-degree relatives with breast cancer: 1

Number of breast biopsies: 2

Race: Black

Estimation of 5-year risk for invasive breast cancer = 2.4%

Estimation of lifetime risk for invasive breast cancer = 13.7%

2. *Julie is a 56-year-old Black female with an estimated 5-year risk of breast cancer equal to 2.4% and lifetime risk equal to 13.7%.*

    a. She has had two benign breast biopsies and one sister with breast cancer.

    b. Julie recently had a total abdominal hysterectomy with bilateral salpingo-oopherectomy due to fibroids. Her gynecologist placed her on HRT following the surgery. She currently denies postmenopausal symptoms but is uncertain how she might feel discontinuing the medication.

    c. She has a history of hypertension that is well controlled.

    d. Julie has three options relative to breast cancer risk reduction.

        i. The HRT may be discontinued and tamoxifen initiated. By taking tamoxifen, Julie will reduce her estimated lifetime risk of breast cancer by 49% in relative terms. There is no risk for endometrial cancer since she has had a hysterectomy. The risk of a thromboembolic event will be no greater than that with HRT. Postmenopausal symptoms may impact Julie's quality of life; however, nonhormonal therapies may be employed. While taking the tamoxifen, she may also be protected against bone loss.

        ii. Julie may choose to continue HRT in combination with close clinical follow-up for breast cancer screening. With the continuation of HRT, she will be increasing her risk for breast cancer. She may benefit, however, from the prevention of osteoporosis and management of postmenopausal symptoms. As with tamoxifen, HRT carries a threefold increased risk for thromboembolitic events.

iii. Finally, she may choose to stop the HRT without initiating tamoxifen for risk reduction. By doing so, she will reduce the risk of breast cancer development associated with estrogen use. Julie will also reduce her risk for thromboembolitic events. She will be more prone to bone loss and postmenopausal symptoms.

Sue

Patient age: 42

Age at first period: 12

Age at first birth: 21

Number of first-degree relatives with breast cancer: 1

Number of breast biopsies: 1

Any biopsies showing hyperplasia: Yes

Race: White

Estimation of 5-year risk for invasive breast cancer = 3.9%

Estimation of lifetime risk for invasive breast cancer = 37.5%

---

3. Sue is a 42-year-old mother with an estimated 5-year risk of breast cancer equal to 3.9%. Her lifetime risk equals 37.5%.

a. Sue is anxious because her mother had breast cancer, and she recently had an excisional biopsy of the right breast that revealed atypical ductal hyperplasia.

b. She is interested in risk reduction strategies.

c. In her history, it is noted that Sue has two children and had a tubal ligation during her last C-section.

d. Sue is an optimal candidate for tamoxifen for the following reasons:

   i. Given her history of atypical hyperplasia, tamoxifen therapy will reduce her estimated lifetime risk for invasive breast cancer by 86%.

   ii. Although she has not had a hysterectomy, the occurrence of endometrial cancer in women less than 50 years of age was not increased by tamoxifen in the Breast Cancer Prevention Trial.[2]

   iii. Additionally, Sue has no further plans for having children, and her tubal ligation provides excellent nonhormonal contraception while taking tamoxifen.

B. Symptom management (see also Chapters 7 and 8)

1. When the decision is made to start tamoxifen, a partnership is established between the patient and the health care provider who prescribes the medication.

2. The goal is to manage the patient through five years of therapy at a dose of 20 mg daily while minimizing side effects and complications.

TABLE 10.4	Management of Hot Flashes

Over-the-Counter Products	Prescription Medications

• Vitamin E 400–800 U/daily
• Evening Primrose Oil
  1–2 capsules up to three
  times daily
• Vitamin B Complex 200 mg/daily
• Peridin-C 2 tablets/three times daily
  (Vitamin C plus bioflavonoids)
	• Effexor XR 37.5–75 mg/daily
	• Paxil 10 mg/daily × 1 week
	  Then 20 mg/daily
	
	• Bellamine S one tablet twice daily
	• Clonidine (Catapres)
	  0.05 mg twice daily, may increase
	  to 0.1 mg twice daily
	  Patch: 0.1 mg/weekly

3. *Educating the patient is a key component of the management strategy. Reinforce the need for communication regarding concerns, potential problems, and change in health status.*

4. *A number of the side effects women experience while taking tamoxifen may be managed using over-the-counter products or prescription medications. Nonpharmacologic approaches may also be employed.*

5. *Management of hot flashes.*

   a. Lifestyle modifications, over-the-counter products (OTC), and prescription medications may be initiated alone or in combination to reduce or alleviate vasomotor symptoms. Specific dosing recommendations for OTC products and prescription medications are outlined in Table 10.4.

   b. General guidelines for using nonhormonal agents to control hot flashes:
      i. Initiate lifestyle modifications and OTC agents first.
      ii. Allow at least 4 to 6 weeks for the interventions to work.
      iii. Add only one intervention at a time.
      iv. OTC agents may be used in combination with one another, but only one prescription agent should be used at any given time.
      v. Women may be on an OTC agent and a prescription agent at the same time.
      vi. A brief drug holiday from tamoxifen may be necessary and beneficial if symptoms persist without relief.

   c. Lifestyle modifications.[15]
      i. Dress in layers, removing clothing as needed.
      ii. Wear breathable fabric such as cotton, linen, or rayon.
      iii. Wear cotton nightclothes and use cotton bed linens.
      iv. Keep ice water handy and sip as needed.
      v. Avoid triggers such as alcohol, caffeine, spicy foods, hot foods, diet pills, smoking, hot showers, hot tubs, saunas, and hot weather.
      vi. Exercise regularly.
      vii. Manage stress and incorporate relaxation techniques into daily activities.
      viii. Eat a diet low in fat.

    d. Over-the-counter medications.

        i. Vitamin E.[16]

        ii. Evening primrose oil.[17]

        iii. Vitamin B complex.[18]

        iv. Vitamin C plus bioflavinoids (Periden-C).[18]

        v. Although a popular alternative to HRT, the safety of herbal agents containing phytoestrogens is not known. Women should be cautioned regarding their use.

    e. Pharmocologic agents.

        i. Effexor® (venlafaxine hydrochloride)

- This pharmacologic agent is proven effective in reducing hot flashes by 50% in women with a personal history of breast cancer.[19]
- First-line pharmcologic agent as the side effects associated with Effexor® are minimal.
- The antidepressant properties prove especially helpful in women experiencing irritability or moodiness.

        ii. Paxil® (paroxetine hydrochloride)

- An alternative for women unable to tolerate Effexor®
- Reduces the frequency and severity of hot flashes by 67% and 75%, respectively, in breast cancer survivors[20]

        iii. Bellamine-S® (Phenobarbital-belladonna-ergotamine)[18]

- Helpful for women with problems sleeping or experiencing nighttime hot flashes
- Limited by daytime sedation if dosing twice daily as recommended

        iv. Clonidine (Catapres®)[21,22]

- Controls the vascular response to the brain's command to give off heat quickly
- May be especially helpful in women with hypertension

6. *Management of vaginal dryness.*

    a. Vaginal dryness with associated dyspurenia can adversely affect quality of life. The implementation of nonhormonal OTC products or appropriate hormonal agents may significantly reduce discomfort.

    b. Estring®.[23]

        i. Estring® vaginal ring provides relief of vaginal dryness by emitting 7.5 mcg estradiol to the vaginal mucosa over a 24-hour period.

        ii. The ring is placed in the upper third of the vaginal vault by the patient. It remains in place for 90 days.

        iii. Placement of Estring® in the vagina results in a rapid rise in estradiol levels in the bloodstream. Within 24 hours, the estradiol levels return to baseline.

        iv. The woman is able to swim, exercise, bathe, or have intercourse without removal.

        v. Estring® use may be problematic in women with uterine prolapse unless a pessary effect is achieved. This is uncommon as the ring is quite small and pliable.

        vi. Estring® is not effective in alleviating systemic symptoms of menopause (e.g., hot flashes).

    c. Vagifem®.[23]

        i. Vaginal tablet containing 25 mcg of estradiol.

        ii. Indicated for the treatment of atrophic vaginitis.

        iii. Recommended dose is one tablet intravaginally at bedtime ×2 weeks then reduce dose to one tablet twice weekly.

    d. Over-the-counter products.
      i. Vaginal lubricants such as Astroglide® or Replens® may be used. It is recommended that these products be used as needed, up to several times daily, to maintain vaginal moisture.
      ii. K–Y Jelly is recommended before intercourse.
      iii. Acidophilus 460 mg daily may also prove helpful.

7. *Leg cramps.*
    a. Leg cramps are a rare side effect of tamoxifen.
    b. Encourage exercise.
    c. Encourage a healthy diet high in calcium and potassium.
    d. Calcium or calcium/magnesium supplements are available OTC.
    e. Tonic water, which contains a limited amount of quinine, may provide relief from the discomfort of leg cramps. Tonic water may be taken alone or in combination with juice or tap water.

8. *Weight gain.*
    a. Although perceived as a side effect of tamoxifen, in BCPT, there was no significant difference in weight gain when comparing the tamoxifen and placebo groups.
    b. If the patient perceives weight gain as an annoying side effect of the drug, encourage her to exercise and eat a healthy diet.
    c. Consultation with a dietician may be helpful.
    d. Thyroid function tests may be considered.

9. *Depression: BCPT demonstrated no significant difference in the incidence of depression between the placebo and the treatment groups.*[14]

C. Follow-up recommendations

1. *Perform clinical breast examination every six months and annual mammography.*

2. *Encourage annual gynecologic examinations in women with uterus.*

3. *Instruct the patient to report any abnormal uterine bleeding immediately. The American College of Obstetrics and Gynecology (ACOG) recommendations for monitoring women taking tamoxifen are available in Table 10.5. Perform pelvic ultrasound and endometrial biopsy as indicated.*[24]

TABLE 10.5	**ACOG Recommendations for Monitoring Women on Tamoxifen for Endometrial Pathology**

1. Annual gynecologic evaluation.
2. Routine biopsy and ultrasound *not* necessary in absence of symptoms.
3. Alert patients to the signs of endometrial pathology.
4. Instruct patients to report abnormal vaginal bleeding.
5. Endometrial sampling and gynecologic evaluation in the presence of abnormal uterine bleeding.
6. If atypical endometrial hyperplasia develops, appropriate gynecologic management should be initiated and tamoxifen use should be reassessed.

ACOG Committee on Gynecologic Practice, April 2000.

4. *At each follow-up visit, educate patients and question them about:*
   a. Breast symptoms
   b. Gynecological symptoms (if uterus intact), reminding women to report any abnormal vaginal bleeding immediately
   c. Thromboembolic symptoms
      i. Lower extremity pain, erythema, or swelling.
      ii. Chest pain or dyspnea.
      iii. Muscle weakness, facial drooping, or inability to speak.
      iv. Instruct the patient to report acute onset of symptoms immediately.
5. *Encourage monthly breast self-examination.*

VI. Conclusions

Being aware of the current guidelines for breast cancer prevention and risk reduction is a daunting task. If approached systematically, however, the healthcare provider will be able to determine a woman's specific risk and individualize a plan of care by incorporating the appropriate risk reduction strategies.

References

1. Daly M. NCCN Practice Guidelines: genetics/familial high-risk cancer screening. *Oncology* 1999;13:161–183.

2. Fisher B, Costantino JP, Wickerham DL, et al. Tamoxifen for prevention of breast cancer: report of the National Surgical Adjuvant Breast and Bowel Project P–1 Study. *J Natl Cancer Inst* 1998;90:1371–1388.

3. National Cancer Institute. Cancer New Web site. Available at: http:/www.cancernet.nci.nih.gov. Accessed January 2002.

4. Bevers TB. Primary prevention of breast cancer and screening for early detection of breast cancer. In: Hunt KK, Robb GL, Strom EA, et al., eds. *M. D. Anderson Cancer Care Series: Breast Cancer.* New York: Springer-Verlag; 2001:20–47.

5. Dooley WC, Ljung BM, Veronesi U. Ductal lavage for detection of cellular atypia in women at high risk for breast cancer. *J Natl Cancer Inst* 2001;93,1624–1632.

6. American Cancer Society. *Breast Cancer Facts & Figures, 2001–2002.* Atlanta, GA: American Cancer Society; 2001;1–23.

7 Feuer EJ, Wun LM, Boring CC, Flanders WD, Timmel MJ, Tong T. The lifetime risk of developing breast cancer. *J Natl Cancer Inst* 1993;85:892–897.

8. Breast Screening Practice Guidelines. NCCN: Version 1.2001.

9. King MC, Wieand S, Hale K, et al. Tamoxifen and breast cancer incidence among women with inherited mutations in BRCA1 and BRCA2. *JAMA* 2001;286:2251–2256.

10. Lippman SM, Brown PH. Tamoxifen prevention of breast cancer: an instance of the fingerpost. *J Natl Cancer Inst* 1999;91:1809–1819.

11. Chlebowski R, Col N, Weiner E, et al., for the ASCO Breast Cancer Technology Assessment Working Group. American society of clinical oncology technology assessment of pharmacologic interventions for breast cancer risk reduction including tamoxifen, raloxifene, and aromatase inhibition. *J Clin Oncol* 2002;20:3328–3343.

12. Gail MH, Costantino JP, Bryant J, et al. Weighing the risks and benefits of tamoxifen treatment for preventing breast cancer. *J Natl Cancer Inst* 1999;91:1829–1846.

13. Day R, Ganz PA, Costantino JP, et al. Health-related quality of life and tamoxifen in breast cancer prevention: a report from the National Surgical Adjuvant Breast and Bowel Project P–1 Study. *J Clin Oncol* 1999;17:2659.

14. Day R, Ganz PA, Costantino JP. Tamoxifen and depression: more evidence from the National Surgical Adjuvant Breast and Bowel Project's Breast Cancer Prevention (P–1) Randomized Study. *J Natl Cancer Inst* 2001;93:1615–1623.

15. Lucero MA, McCloskey WW. Alternatives to estrogen for the treatment of hot flashes. *Ann Pharmacother* 1997;31:915–917.

16. Barton DL, Loprinzi CL, Quella SK, et al. Prospective evaluation of vitamin E for hot flashes in breast cancer survivors. *J Clin Oncol* 1998;16:495–500.

17. Gruenwald J, Brendler T, Jaenicke C, eds. *PDR for Herbal Medicines.* Montvale, NJ: Medical Economics Company; 1998:998–999.

18 National Surgical Adjuvant Breast and Bowel Project. The study of tamoxifen and raloxifene (STAR). Available at: www.nsabp.pitt.edu. Accessed January 2002.

19. Loprinzi CL, Pisansky RF, Sloan JA, et al. Pilot evaluation of venlafaxine hydrochloride for the therapy of hot flashes in cancer survivors. *J Clin Oncol* 1998;16:2377–2381.

20. Stearns V, Isaacs C, Rowland J, et al. A pilot trial assessing the efficacy of paroxetine hydrochloride (Paxil®) in controlling hot flashes in breast cancer survivors. *Ann Oncol* 2000;11:17–22.

21. Pandya KJ, Raubertas RF, Flynn PJ, et al. Oral clonidine in postmenopausal patients with breast cancer experiencing tamoxifen-induced hot flashes: a University of Rochester Cancer Center Community Clinical Oncology Program Study. *Ann Intern Med* 2000;132:788–793.

22. Goldberg RM, Loprinzi CL, O'Fallon JR, et al. Transdermal clonidine for ameliorating tamoxifen induced hot flashes. *J Clin Oncol* 1994;12:155–158.

23. Murray L., Kelly GL, ed. *Physician Desk Reference.* Montvale, NJ: Medical Economics Co; 2002:2811–2814, 2857–2860.

24. ACOG committee opinion. Tamoxifen and endometrial cancer. *Int J Obstet Gynecol* 2001;73:77–79.

chapter 11

Counseling about the Genetics of Breast Cancer

Paula Trahan Rieger, RN, MSN, CS, AOCN®, FAAN
Director, International Affairs
American Society of Clinical Oncology
formerly:
Nurse Practitioner, Clinical Cancer Prevention
Human Clinical Cancer Genetics
The University of Texas M.D. Anderson Cancer Center
Houston, TX

I. **Definition and Standards of Cancer Genetic Counseling**[1–3]

   A. A risk assessment, communication, and educational process by which individuals and family members receive information about:

      1. *The risk for developing cancer;*

      2. *Strategies for managing an increased risk for developing cancer;*

      3. *The nature and limitations of genetic tests, benefits, risks, and costs of genetic testing; and*

      4. *The meaning of test results.*

   B. The goal is to have individuals and families learn and understand aspects of genetics that have an impact upon their risk for developing cancer, to make informed health decisions, and to receive support in integrating personal and family genetic information into their lives.

   C. Individuals must receive adequate information to make informed decisions concerning their health and must be able to give informed consent to undergo testing as appropriate.

   D. Genetic testing should be conducted only in conjunction with cancer genetic counseling.

II. **Cancer Genetic Counseling Process**[4–12]

   A. Information in this section is presented at the level that it would be presented to the patient.

   B. Assessment and information gathering.

      1. *Determination of the reason for referral*

         a. Patient generated referral

            i. Common reasons patients may seek cancer genetic counseling:

- To obtain information about their risk of developing cancer
- To obtain information about their risk for developing additional cancers
- To determine strategies for managing the risk of developing cancer
- To obtain information for other family members
- To obtain cancer genetic testing

         b. Physician or provider generated referral

            i. Common reasons include:

- Recognition of characteristics of a hereditary cancer syndrome (see Table 11.1)
- To obtain input on a risk management plan

TABLE 11.1	Characteristics Suggestive of the Presence of a Cancer Predisposition Gene in a Family Pedigree

Increased number of cancers
Unexpectedly early age of onset of tumors
Multiple tumors in a single individual
Rare tumors
Identifiable pattern of cancers predictive of a cancer syndrome
Nonmalignant manifestations of a cancer gene syndrome
Ethnic background or "founder" effects

- To have a patient obtain cancer genetic testing
- Patient request

2. *Information gathering*

   a. Family history.[13,14]

      i. Collect information on three generations when possible, including parents, siblings, aunts, uncles, and grandparents at a minimum.

      ii. It is important to collect both maternal and paternal histories. As complete a picture as possible of the family should be obtained, including whether family members are still living or have died. Information on those family members who are living and unaffected with cancer is as important as that for those who have had a diagnosis of cancer.

      iii. Information on cancers in family members should include:

         - The type of cancer.
         - Age at diagnosis.
         - Age at death.
         - Bilaterality (e.g., two primary breast tumors).
         - Pathology (e.g., is the cancer *in situ* or invasive).
         - The presence of more than one primary tumor (e.g., a person with colon and uterine cancer or breast cancer and ovarian cancer).
         - When providing family cancer history, patients may not always be able to distinguish between a metastatic tumor and a second primary tumor.

      iv. Information is generally best collected prior to the visit through the use of a family history questionnaire or a telephone interview.

      v. Family history is depicted in a pedigree (visual representation of the family history) so that it can easily be reviewed with the patient (see Figure 11.1) and used, where appropriate, to share the information with other health care practitioners such as genetic counselors, nurse practitioners, or consulting physicians.

         - Pedigrees may be hand drawn.
         - Computerized programs are available for the generation of pedigrees (e.g., Cyrillic, Prodigy).

      vi. Verification of cancers reported in the family is necessary as inherited forms of cancer are recognized almost solely on the basis of family history. This is done either through pathology reports or death certificates. Permission is required to obtain medical records.

         - Ovarian cancer is often confused with other female and abdominal cancers. Verification is important because the presence of an ovarian cancer will significantly increase the probability of testing positive for a mutation in either the BRCA1 or BRCA2 gene.
         - Research has shown that, in general, reports of breast cancer within the family are reliable.
         - Information must be obtained with signed permission of the person or living next of kin. It is helpful to have forms available for patients and families to use in this process.

      vii. Determine if genetic testing has been done, on which family member it was done, and whether results are available.

FIGURE 11.1 Pedigree depicting a family history of breast cancer

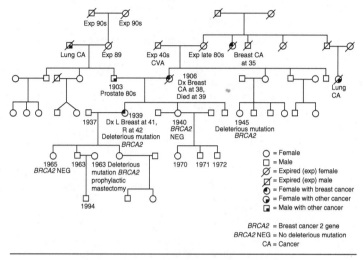

Rieger, PT. In: Yarbro CH, Hansen Frogge M, Goodman M, Groenwald SL, eds. *Cancer Nursing: Principles and Practice.* 5th ed. Sudbury, MA: Jones & Bartlett Publishers; 2000:192.

b. Personal history.[15]
   i. Obtain past medical history and screening practices.
      • Determine results of screening tests.
      • Determine the frequency at which screening was done and the age it was initiated.
      • Determine where screening is currently being performed and by whom.
      • Ascertain the subject's knowledge concerning self-examination (e.g., breast self exam).
   ii. History relevant to breast cancer risk such as:
      • Age of menarche
      • Age of first live birth
      • Number of breast biopsies
   iii. Lifestyle information, including:
      • Smoking history
      • Diet
      • Alcohol intake
      • Exercise
   iv. For patients who already have a diagnosis of cancer, obtain information on the:
      • Diagnosis
      • Age at diagnosis
      • Pathology
      • Treatment course

    c. Patient perception of risk for developing cancer.[16]
      i. Research has shown and clinical practice has substantiated that patients with a family history of cancer often overestimate their risk for developing cancer to a significant degree.
      ii. Most patients will state that they have a 50% or greater lifetime risk of developing breast cancer, with many verbalizing a 75% or greater lifetime risk. A risk this high would only be seen in those individuals who carry a mutation in currently identified genes that predispose for the development of cancer, such as the BRCA1 or BRCA2 gene.
      iii. Often women are very anxious about their risk of developing a breast cancer. It is important to take time to discuss:
- Their concerns
- Their feelings and emotions associated with the cancers that have occurred in their family
- Their fears and concerns about themselves

      iv. Determine the patient's beliefs about cancer and its causation. Patients often believe there is something "hereditary" in their family that is responsible for the cancers.

    d. Evaluate the patient's knowledge about cancer, hereditary cancers, and cancer genetic testing.
      i. This is often most easily accomplished with an open-ended question to allow the patient to express what they know and understand.
      ii. Determine where have they obtained the information they have.
      iii. Determine what questions they have, if any.

    e. Social and cultural concerns.
      i. Assess social support systems and family relationships because genetic information will have relevance and potential impact upon family members.
      ii. Cultural heritage and any specific beliefs related to cancer, hereditary cancer syndromes, or genetic testing should also be identified.

C. Evaluation and analysis of data.

1. *Family and personal history should be reviewed for characteristics of a hereditary cancer syndrome (see Table 11.1).*

2. *Appropriate models should be used (e.g., Gail, Claus, or BRCAPRO) to determine the risk of developing cancer and to determine the probability that the patient or an affected family member would test positive for an alteration in the BRCA1 or BRCA2 gene (e.g., BRCAPRO). For further information on how this is done see Chapter 3.[17]*

3. *Determine the need for additional information to fully evaluate the family (e.g., precise pathologic diagnosis or more adequate recounting of the family history).*

4. *Perform a focused physical examination (e.g., breast exam) if physical examination is part of the services provided. In some centers, only counseling may be provided.*

D. Communication of genetic and risk information.

1. *Provide an overview of the biological basis of cancer and the relationship of risk factors to the development of cancer.*
   a. Discuss the stepwise process of cancer development.
      i. Cancer begins with a mutation in a single cell.
      ii. This mutation is passed along to the progeny of that cell as it replicates.
      iii. Over time, additional mutations may occur.
      iv. After the accumulation of perhaps 5 to 10 mutations, this group of cells may be diagnosed as cancer.
      v. This process takes time (approximately 5 to 10 years) or in some cases, even longer.
      vi. These mutations occur in specific classes of genes known as oncogenes, tumor suppressor genes, and "caretaker" genes.
      vii. The use of diagrams can be extremely helpful to visually represent the process.
   b. Discuss how somatic mutations differ from hereditary mutations.
      i. Somatic mutations occur in body cells. These mutations cannot be passed on to children.
      ii. Hereditary mutations are carried in the germline and may be passed from a parent to their children.
   c. Discuss differences between sporadic cancers, familial cancers, and hereditary cancers.
      i. The majority of cancers in the population occur by random chance and are known as sporadic cancers. For example, one in eight women in their lifetime will develop breast cancer. Explain how risk factors are associated with sporadic cancers (see Chapter 1).
      ii. In familial cancers, there may be a clustering of similar cancers; however, these families do not exhibit the characteristics of a hereditary cancer syndrome. For example, there may be several breast cancers in a family that occur at older ages.
      iii. In familial cancer, risk is increased over that of the population, but not to the degree it is in a hereditary cancer syndrome.
      iv. In hereditary cancer syndromes, specific characteristics are seen, as described in Table 11.1. Individuals who have inherited a genetic alteration in a gene known to be associated with a specific hereditary cancer syndrome are at a greatly increased lifetime risk of developing one of the cancers associated with that syndrome.

2. *Discuss the family cancer history.*
   a. Give an overview of characteristics of the hereditary cancer syndrome and the presence or absence in a patient's family.
   b. Explain the types of cancers and any unique clustering seen in the family.
   c. Explain the degree to which a hereditary cancer syndrome is suspected and which syndrome (e.g., Hereditary breast/Ovarian Cancer syndrome, Li Fraumeni).[18]
   d. Discuss the probability of testing positive for an alteration in either the BRCA1 or BRCA2 gene or other hereditary cancer syndromes that would predispose to breast cancer.

  e. If family history is not indicative of a hereditary cancer syndrome, explain how patient's risk would be calculated (e.g., either familial or sporadic).

3. *Discuss inheritance patterns.*

  a. Define a germline mutation (e.g., a mutation that is carried in either the egg or sperm cells) and explain that cancer predisposition genes are transmitted in an autosomal dominant fashion.

   i. In autosomal dominant patterns of transmission, there is a 50% probability that a parent will pass a genetic mutation to a child.

   ii. Each of us carries two copies of every gene.

   iii. If one copy is altered or mutated and is carried in the germline, then a parent can pass either the good copy or the altered copy to each child they have.

   iv. The probability that a parent with an alteration in a cancer predisposition gene, such as BRCA1 or BRCA2, would pass that alteration on to their children is 50% for each child.

4. *Discuss risk for developing cancer.*

  a. Review population risk for developing a breast cancer (e.g., one in eight women will develop a breast cancer) and how the patient's risk may differ depending on personal and family history and other relevant risk factors.

  b. Explain which models were used to determine risk and the strengths and limitations of those models (see Chapter 3).

  c. Present risk information in a way that is understandable for the patient. For example, it is often easier for patients to understand that they carry a 30% cumulative lifetime risk of developing a breast cancer than a fivefold relative risk.

  d. It is important to review the risk of developing an additional cancer that may be associated with a hereditary cancer syndrome such as ovarian cancer or for developing a second breast cancer, in women who have already been diagnosed with a breast cancer.

  e. It is important to discuss that even if there is a hereditary cancer syndrome in the family and the patient inherits the alteration known to be present in the family that the risk for developing cancer is not 100%.

   i. Review again the stepwise process of cancer development

   ii. Being born with a mutation in BRCA1, for example, is like being born with one strike against you.

   iii. Other mutations must occur before a cancer ultimately develops.

   iv. Some may never develop a cancer even though they have inherited an alteration.

   v. This is why BRCA1 and BRCA2 are called cancer predisposition genes. For those that inherit an alteration in one of these genes, they are predisposed to an increased risk of specific cancers (e.g., primarily breast and ovarian cancer) in their lifetime.

5. *Discuss the ramifications and appropriateness of cancer predisposition genetic testing.*

  a. If genetic testing were done on an affected family member (e.g., one who has developed a cancer), provide and discuss an estimate regarding the probability that a positive (deleterious) result would be found. (See Chapter 3 for a discussion of models used in genetic risk assessment.)

   b. If the patient has breast or ovarian cancer, they would carry the same estimate.

   c. If the patient does not have a cancer, then the probability that they would carry the alteration is decreased depending on their position in the pedigree.

      i. For example, if the patient's mother has breast cancer and the patient does not, then there is a 50% probability that the patient would have inherited a genetic alteration from her mother. The probability that the family would test positive is cut by 50% for the patient if they were the person to undergo testing.

      ii. If the breast cancer tracks on the paternal side of the family, the estimate for the patient drops to 25%. There is a 50% probability that the patient's father would have inherited the alteration and a 50% probability the father would pass that alteration on to his children.

   d. Review the benefits, risks, and limitations of predictive genetic testing (see section III Genetic Testing).

      i. Review the cost of testing and the issues related to insurer coverage.

      ii. Review the potential answers that may be obtained and how they will affect the patient and the family.

      iii. Review who in the family is the best person to undergo testing and why (e.g., it is always preferable to test a family member who is affected with a cancer first).

      iv. In general, if there is at least a 10% probability that the individual would test positive, it is reasonable to consider testing.

      v. Discuss strategies that will maintain the confidentiality of the test results if the patient so desires.

6. *Discuss strategies for managing increased risk for developing cancer (see Figure 3.2, Chapter 3).*[19–21]

   a. There is no standard of care that relates to the best strategy for managing the increased risk for breast cancer associated with an alteration in a cancer predisposition gene. Recommendations are based largely on expert opinion due to the absence of prospectively validated management strategies.

   b. Developing an appropriate risk management plan involves lengthy and thoughtful discussion between the patient and her healthcare providers.

   c. The provider should offer an overview of the strategies available and the data supporting their efficacy in decreasing risk. The provider should determine which strategies make the patient feel most comfortable in managing her risk.

   d. When possible, patients should enter clinical research trials that are evaluating risk management strategies in patients at an increased risk of developing cancer.

   e. In 1998, the National Cancer Institute (NCI) developed the Cancer Genetics Network (CGN) to conduct systematic, empirical research on issues related to the burgeoning field of cancer genetics and hereditary cancer syndromes.

   f. Eight sites across the country were identified and have been funded (see Table 11.2). Within this network, clinical trials to evaluate the best strategies for managing risk are beginning to emerge.

TABLE 11.2 Cancer Genetics Network Sites

Participating Institutions

Center	Principal Investigators	Collaborators
Carolina-Georgia Cancer Genetics Network Center	Joellen Schildkraut, PhD Duke University Medical Center Durham, NC	Emory University, Atlanta, GA University of North Carolina Chapel Hill, NC
Georgetown University Medical Center's Cancer Genetics Network Center	Claudine Isaacs, MD Georgetown University Lombardi Cancer Center Washington, DC	None
Mid-Atlantic Cancer Genetics Network Center	Constance Griffin, MD Johns Hopkins University, Baltimore, Md	Greater Baltimore Medical Center, Baltimore, MD
Northwest Cancer Genetics Network	John D Potter, MD, PhD Fred Hutchinson Cancer Research Center Seattle, WA	University of Washington School of Medicine Seattle, WA
Rocky Mountain Cancer Genetics Coalition	Geraldine Mineau, PhD, University of Utah Salt Lake City, UT	University of New Mexico, Albuquerque, NM University of Colorado, Aurora, CO
Texas Cancer Genetics Consortium	Louise C Strong, MD, The University of Texas M. D. Anderson Cancer Center Houston, TX	The University of Texas Health Science Center San Antonio, TX University of Texas Southwestern Medical Center Dallas, TX Baylor College of Medicine Houston, TX
University of Pennsylvania Cancer Genetics Network	Barbara Weber, MD, University of Pennsylvania Philadelphia, PA	None

UCI-UCSD Cancer Genetics Network Center	Hoda Anton-Culver, PhD, University of California Irvine, CA	University of California San Diego, CA
Informatics and Information Technology Group	Hoda Anton-Culver, PhD, University of California Irvine, CA	
	Dianne M Finkelstein, PhD, Massachusetts General Hospital Boston, MA	
	Prakash M Nadkarni, PhD, Yale University New Haven, CT	

Note: The Cancer Genetics Network (CGN) is a national Network of centers specializing in the study of inherited predisposition to cancer. The CGN consists of eight centers and an Informatics and Information Technology Group that provide the supporting informatics and logistics infrastructure.

The CGN's web site is: http://epi.grants.cancer.gov/CGN/members.html.

g. There are four key areas that should be discussed as strategies for managing increased risk for developing cancer. These may be used alone or in combination. For a full review of each strategy, please see the relevant chapters within this text.

i. Lifestyle changes: Review healthy lifestyle habits (e.g., weight control, moderate exercise, diets high in fiber and low in fat content, not smoking, and moderate use of alcohol are important to reinforce).

- It may be difficult to determine the degree to which these strategies diminish risk.
- Being able to "do something" may contribute to empowering patients and improving their psychological outlook.

ii. Chemoprevention: Use natural or synthetic chemical agents to reverse, suppress, or prevent progression to invasive cancer.

- Results released by King et al in 2001[22] indicated that the use of tamoxifen in BRCA2 carriers is more effective for decreasing the risk of developing breast cancer than it is in BRCA1 carriers.
- Women who are carriers of an alteration in BRCA1 are more likely to develop estrogen receptor-negative tumors. In the Breast Cancer Prevention Trial, those women who developed breast cancer while on tamoxifen tended to develop estrogen receptor-negative tumors.
- Women who carry BRCA2 mutations and are postmenopausal should be evaluated for enrollment in the Study of Tamoxifen and Raloxifene (STAR).
- Oral contraceptives provide some protection against ovarian cancer, but it is not known definitively whether they also protect against hereditary forms of ovarian cancer.

  Several studies have evaluated the relationship of oral contraceptive use and the development of ovarian cancer in women with mutations in BRCA1 and BRCA2 genes.

  Although one study failed to identify a protective effect,[23] the preponderance of the epidemiological evidence is that oral contraceptives do decrease the incidence of ovarian cancer in these women.

  Prospective trials are needed, but oral contraceptives represent a reasonable step to consider.[24]

iii. Prophylactic surgery: Data are beginning to emerge that support the use of prophylactic surgery to manage risk in women who are carriers of a mutation in either the BRCA1 or BRCA2 gene. (See Chapter 9)

- The degree of risk reduction associated with prophylactic mastectomy or oophorectomy has not yet been fully determined for individuals who carry a mutation that predisposes for breast or ovarian cancer.
- It is clear, nevertheless, that some risk remains following prophylactic surgery. It is important that women who are carriers of an alteration in BRCA1 or BRCA2 understand that they may still develop a breast cancer following prophylactic mastectomy or ovarian cancer following oophorectomy.

- Hartmann and colleagues performed a retrospective study of 639 women with a family history of breast cancer that underwent bilateral prophylactic mastectomy at the Mayo Clinic between 1960 and 1993.[25] Hartmann showed that prophylactic mastectomy was associated with a reduction in the incidence of breast cancer of at least 90 percent. In a small subset of 26 women with proven inherited mutations in either the BRCA1 or BRCA2 gene, none have developed breast cancer with an average 16.1 years follow-up.

  The data indicate that bilateral prophylactic mastectomy yields a significant reduction in breast cancer risk in BRCA1/2 gene mutation carriers, over 90%.[26]

- In July 2001, Meijers-Heijboer and colleagues[27] published results from a prospective study of 139 women with BRCA1 or BRCA2 gene mutations who were enrolled in a breast cancer surveillance program at the Rotterdam Family Cancer Clinic in the Netherlands.

  Seventy-six of the women underwent prophylactic mastectomy, and the other 63 remained under surveillance.

  There were no cases of breast cancer observed after prophylactic mastectomy with a mean follow-up of 2.9 years. There were eight breast cancers in women who had not undergone prophylactic surgery after a mean follow-up of 3 years.

  Although the numbers are small and the follow-up very short, prophylactic bilateral total mastectomy appears to reduce markedly the incidence of breast cancer at three years of follow-up.

- The lifetime risk of ovarian cancer in BRCA gene mutation carriers is estimated to be 10 to 45%, which is more than tenfold that of the 1 to 2% risk in the general population.

- Prophylactic oophorectomy remains a reasonable option for carriers to consider. It is clear, however, that primary peritoneal carcinoma occurs at a higher frequency in BRCA1 and BRCA2 gene mutation carriers and that prophylactic oophorectomy does not prevent primary peritoneal carcinomatosis.

  Several studies that are complicated by a lack of genetic testing or small sample size have suggested that prophylactic oophorectomy decreases the incidence of ovarian cancer (including primary peritoneal carcinomatosis) by between twofold and tenfold.

  Prophylactic oophorectomy not only decreases the incidence of ovarian cancer, but also decreases the incidence of breast cancer by a significant amount in women who are carriers of a BRCA1 gene mutation.[28]

  If the patient is premenopausal, the provider should discuss the pros and cons of hormone replacement therapy and other strategies to decrease risk for development of osteoporosis.

iv. Screening.

- In principle, for those at increased risk, screening is generally initiated at an earlier age than for those in the general population.

TABLE 11.3	Options for Cancer Prevention/Detection in Carriers of BRCA1 and BRCA2 Gene Mutations

Prevention
Consider chemoprevention options.
> Consider the use of tamoxifen to decrease the risk of breast cancer in BRCA2 carriers.
> For women who are BRCA2 carriers and postmenopausal, consider enrollment in the STAR trial.
> Discuss option of entrance into chemoprevention trials.
>> Data indicates that oral contraceptive pills may decrease the risk of ovarian cancer; the impact on breast cancer is unclear.
>> Consider trials with other chemopreventive agents (e.g., the retinoids) that may have efficacy in this population.

Prophylactic Surgery
Discuss options and limitations of prophylactic mastectomy.
> Decision is generally made on a case-by-case basis.
> Review reconstruction options.
> Arrange consult to surgeon and plastic surgeon.
Discuss options and limitations of prophylactic oophorectomy.
>> Decision is generally made on a case-by-case basis.
>> Discussion should include reproductive desires, role of hormone replacement therapy, management of increased risk for osteoporosis and cardiovascular disease, and management of menopausal symptoms.

Screening
Breast Cancer
Instruction in breast self exam
> Initiate training in breast self exam at young adulthood (age 15–18 years)
Clinical breast exam
> Annual or semiannual beginning at age 25 years
Mammography
> Annual beginning at age 25–30 years
> Some clinicians may use 5–10 years before the earliest cancer developed in the family, although mammography would generally not be initiated before age 25 years.
Ovarian Cancer
CA–125 blood level + Transvaginal ultrasound + Pelvic Exam
> Annual or semiannual beginning at age 30–40 years
> Some centers may recommend that ovarian cancer screening occur more toward age 35 or later, as ovarian cancers tend to occur at a later age than breast cancer.

Data from references 19–21

Clinical trials to determine the most appropriate surveillance measures for those carrying mutated cancer susceptibility genes are needed, and the development of a newer and more sensitive screening test remains a high priority.

    h. For an overview of risk management strategies see Table 11.3 for a review of current recommendations for carriers of a mutation in either the BRCA1 or BRCA2 gene.

E. Supportive counseling.[29,30]

    1. *Discussion of patient and family questions and concerns*

        a. The potential risk for children to develop cancer

        b. Discrimination by insurers and employers

    c. The ability to manage risk effectively

    d. How the information will be documented in the medical record

2. *Provision of emotional and social support*[31-34]

    a. It is important to determine the patient's existing coping patterns and support systems.

    b. Teach new coping strategies as required. A coping style of high monitoring has been associated in some studies with a higher degree of anxiety while awaiting test results.

    c. Assist the patient in identifying strategies to share information about risk or genetic testing results with family members.

       i. For example, the patient should ask family members if they wish to know the results of the patient's genetic test.

       ii. The counseling team can also assist the patient in explaining results to family members if the patient and family so wish.

    d. Assist the patient with psychological responses to receiving genetic test results.

       i. Some studies have demonstrated an increase in knowledge following genetic counseling with no increase in anxiety or depression.

       ii. Others have shown increased anxiety related to positive test results.

       iii. Further assessment is required to determine the psychological impact of receiving a genetic test result.

    e. The majority of patients, however, do not express regret over their decision to undergo genetic testing.

F. Follow-up counseling.

1. *A detailed summary letter is generally provided to patients outlining the information reviewed during the visit. Included in the letter is:*

    a. A summary of the family history

    b. Assessment of the risk for developing cancer

    c The probability of testing positive for a mutation in either the BRCA1 or BRCA2 gene

    d. Genetic testing results, when appropriate

    e. Strategies for managing risk

2. *Periodic follow-up visits should be scheduled to reassess the family or to provide the patient with updated information.*

3. *Provide coordination of the patient's care with other healthcare providers (such as the primary oncologists).*

4. *If there is specific information, for example, genetic test results, that the patient wishes to have released to other providers, it is necessary to have signed permission from the patient that provides direction.*

5. *Discuss which family members should receive the information.*

III. **Genetic Testing**

A. It is important that cancer genetic testing occur in conjunction with cancer genetic counseling.

1. *In addition to the areas discussed within the cancer genetic counseling process, the following areas should be covered in reference to genetic testing.*

TABLE 11.4	Factors Influencing Cancer Genetic Counseling

Individual Frame of Reference
  Personal philosophy about cancer
  Life experience with cancer
  Self-perception of risk
  Anxiety over cancer risk
  Opinions about obtaining genetic information
Family Considerations
  Differing opinions about obtaining genetic information
  Presence of family members during counseling
Cultural and Ethnic
  Views on cancer as a disease
  Views on genetics and genetic testing
  Decision-making process within the family
Structural
  Healthcare providers
    Team mix providing counseling and expertise in cancer care
  Setting
    Wellness setting—e.g., prevention center
    Illness setting—e.g., within cancer treatment center
  Payment for counseling services
  Payment for genetic testing
  Timing (e.g., near recent diagnosis of cancer, near recent death in the
  family from cancer)
  Recordkeeping
    Documentation of services
    Communication with other healthcare professionals

    2. *In the broadest sense, genetic tests are defined as the analysis of human DNA, RNA, chromosomes, proteins, and other gene products to detect disease-related genotypes, mutations, phenotypes, or karyotypes.*

  B. Setting for testing.

    1. *The provision of cancer genetic counseling may be impacted by many factors. Table 11.4 outlines individual, family, cultural, ethnic, and structural factors that must be considered when providing services.*

    2. *Many centers only offer cancer genetic testing within the context of a clinical research trial.*

    3. *Genetic testing for mutations in the BRCA1 or BRCA2 genes is commercially available and is offered within the community setting outside of a cancer research center.*

    4. *The American Society of Clinical Oncology initially set forth a statement on cancer predisposition testing in 1996.[35] General principles for cancer genetic testing that would apply to genetic testing for BRCA1 or BRCA2 mutations are as follows:*

      a. The person has individual or a strong family history suggestive of genetic etiology;

      b. The test can be adequately interpreted; and

      c. The results will influence the medical management of the patient or family member.

      d. As of August 2002, this statement is in the process of revision.

TABLE 11.5	National Comprehensive Cancer Network Criteria for Hereditary Breast/Ovarian Cancer Syndrome

Member of a known BRCA1/BRCA2 family

Personal history of breast cancer and one or more of the following:
Diagnosed at age 40 years or less, with or without family history
Diagnosed at age 50 years or less or with bilateral breast cancer, **with**

      One or more close relatives with breast cancer
or   One or more close relatives with ovarian cancer
Diagnosed at any age, **with**

      Two or more close relatives with ovarian cancer at any age **or**
      Two or more relatives with breast cancer, especially if one or more
      women are diagnosed before age 50 or have bilateral disease
      Close male relative with breast cancer
      Of Ashkenazi Jewish heritage and diagnosed at age 50 years or less,
      no additional family history required

or
Of Ashkenazi Jewish heritage and diagnosed at any age if family history of
breast and/or ovarian cancer

Personal history of ovarian cancer
One or more close relatives with ovarian cancer
One or more close female relatives with breast cancer at age 50 years or less,
or with bilateral breast cancer
Two or more close relatives with breast cancer
One or more close male relatives with breast cancer
Of Ashkenazi Jewish heritage, no additional family history required

Male breast cancer: personal or family history
One or more close male relatives with breast cancer
One or more close female relatives with breast or ovarian cancer

Family history only
One or more close relatives with breast cancer at age 40 years or less **or**
with bilateral breast cancer
Two or more close relatives with ovarian cancer
Two or more close relatives with breast cancer, especially if one or more
relatives was diagnosed at age 50 years or less
One or more close relatives with breast cancer, and one or more relatives
with ovarian cancer
Of Ashkenazi Jewish heritage, with one close relative with breast or ovarian
cancer

Data from references 20–21

    5. *The determination of a qualified healthcare professional directly involved in the care of the individual being tested should be relied upon in making determinations of the appropriateness of genetic testing.*
    6. *Criteria for testing have also been developed by the National Comprehensive Cancer Network (NCCN) (see Table 11.5).[21]*
  C. Informed consent.[36–38]
    1. *Several organizations have developed position statements on cancer genetic testing. All are in agreement that a process of informed consent must occur. Many recommend that the patient sign a written informed consent document to undergo cancer genetic testing.*

2. Topics that should be reviewed during the process of informed consent include:
   a. The purpose of the genetic test
   b. The reason for offering testing
   c. The type and nature of the genetic condition being tested for
   d. The accuracy of the genetic test
   e. The benefits of participating in testing
   f. The risks associated with genetic testing, including unexpected results
   g. Other available testing options
   h. Available treatment and intervention options
   i. Further decision making that may be needed on receipt of test results
   j. Consent to use patient's DNA for further research purposes if applicable
   k. Availability of additional counseling and support services
   l. Acknowledgment of the right to not undergo testing or to not receive test results

D. Accuracy of the test and interpretation of results.[39]

1. Information about cancer predisposition testing abounds in the lay media and on the Internet. Individuals frequently seek predisposition testing with unrealistic expectations of what testing can provide.

2. During cancer genetic counseling, the healthcare professional providing counseling must review:
   a. How the test is performed
   b. The type of test to be used (e.g., protein truncation versus full sequencing of the gene)
   c. The sensitivity and specificity of the test
   d. Who in the family is the best person to test (e.g., one who has already developed a cancer associated with the syndrome)
   e. Potential answers that may be obtained
   f. The meaning of each answer

3. Commercially available genetic tests are based on a variety of techniques such as protein truncation assays, heteroduplex analysis, versions of single-strand conformational polymorphism (SSCP) analysis, and direct sequencing of the gene of interest.

4. The cost of commercial genetic predisposition testing may range from several hundred dollars (e.g., when confirming a known mutation that has been found in another family member or when using panels that assess several mutations commonly seen in those of a specific heritage) to several thousand dollars for full sequencing of large genes such as BRCA1 or BRCA2.[40]

5. There is one commercial laboratory in the United States that currently provides genetic testing for alterations in BRCA1 or BRCA2. Myriad Genetic Laboratories is located in Salt Lake City, Utah.

6. Clinicians can obtain information about laboratories that offer genetic testing through www.genetests.org. This site provides a national directory of DNA diagnostic laboratories and is designed for health care providers. Registration is required.

7. Depending on the test being performed and the approach being used, it often requires 4 to 6 weeks to obtain test results.

8. Testing for alterations in the BRCA1 or BRCA2 genes by Myriad Genetic Laboratories is generally done with the use of a blood sample.

9. For testing of other genes associated with rare hereditary cancer syndromes such as the PTEN gene for Cowden's disease, clinicians should consult the specific laboratory.

10. Possible test results

   a. Deleterious mutation (positive test result)—The individual must understand clearly that this denotes a predisposition for the development of cancer, not a diagnosis or even the inevitability of cancer development.

   b. Information related to the penetrance of the mutation must be reviewed. (See Chapter 3 on breast cancer genetics.)

   c. Negative test result (in the presence of a known mutation in the family)—When there is a known mutation in the family and an individual's test is negative for that mutation, it is important for the individual to realize that he or she still has the general population risk for the development of cancer.

   d. Negative test result—A negative test result is often difficult to interpret when no known mutation has yet been detected in a family. Negative test results may be obtained because:

      i. The test used missed something (i.e., a false negative because of technical difficulties or the location of a mutation in a region of the gene not tested, such as promoter, enhancer, or intronic regions);

      ii. There is not as yet an undiscovered gene responsible for the constellation of cancers seen in the family; or

      iii. The cancers may have resulted purely from chance.

      iv. An estimate of the patient's risk for developing cancer and management strategies for such risk remain determined by the patient's personal and family history.

   e. Inconclusive results—If sequence changes are found about which insufficient information exists to determine whether the changes are deleterious or simply a harmless genetic variation within the population (polymorphism), the result is termed inconclusive. In such cases, it remains difficult to determine cancer risk. This would be determined, however, based on the patient's personal and family history.

11. To provide the most complete information for a family, it is best to test an affected individual (e.g., one who has already developed a cancer associated with the syndrome).

    a. Some centers will offer testing only to affected individuals.

    b. Some centers may not test a child before the parents because test results will have implications for the parents.

12. Following disclosure of test results, management strategies should be reviewed at length with the patient (see section on risk management and relevant chapters).

13. In the instance of a positive test result, referral for consultation with a surgeon for discussion of prophylactic surgery, or to a specialized screening clinic, or for consideration for clinical trials that are evaluating risk

management strategies (e.g., chemoprevention, cancer detection strategies) should be considered.

14. Historically, the genetic counseling process has been based on the premise of using a nondirective approach.

15. With respect to cancer genetic counseling, recommendations should be made for cancer screening.

   a. At this time, there is no standard of practice with respect to the best strategy for managing risk in a patient known to be a carrier of a BRCA1 or BRCA2 gene mutation.

   b. The patient and her or his clinician must select the strategy that makes them most comfortable in managing risk.

   c. This often requires lengthy discussion between the patient and the healthcare provider.

16. Those providing counseling services should be aware of their own biases and philosophy toward testing so that their opinions do not inadvertently or unnecessarily influence those of the patient.

E. Confidentiality of test results.

   1. The confidentiality of results remains an area of concern. Many individuals harbor fears about the potential misuse of information or negative sequelae that may result from release of test results. Concerns include:

      a. Discrimination by insurers

      b. Discrimination by employers

      c. Discrimination for licensure examinations

      d. Concern over release to other family members

   2. Many states have now enacted legislation prohibiting discrimination by health insurers. Legislation in some states also covers discrimination by employers.

   3. Federal legislation passed in 1996, the Kennedy-Kassebaum bill, includes safeguards against discrimination based on genetic information. Its effectiveness in protecting consumers has yet to be tested in the courts.

   4. The Americans with Disabilities Act (ADA) also offers some protections, although this has not yet been sufficiently tested through case law.

   5. During the 107th United States Congress, there were several bills related to protection against genetic discrimination under consideration.

   6. To date, few if any cases of overt discrimination related to cancer genetic testing have been documented.

   7. Consideration must be given to how results are documented, communicated, and managed in the clinical setting to ensure confidentiality. The standard used in any clinical setting should be reviewed with the patient.

      a. For example, in some centers, the patient's test results may not be placed in the primary medical record.

      b. Signed permission should be obtained from the patient before providing test results to other healthcare providers.

   8. See Table 11.6 for a list of benefits and risks of genetic testing that should be reviewed with the patient.

TABLE 11.6   Benefits and Risks of Cancer Genetic Testing

Positive Results	Inconclusive Results	Negative Results*
Benefits	**Benefits**	**Benefits**
Ability to tailor more aggressive cancer screening and detection measures to those individuals carrying the highest risk	May provide feeling of empowerment, i.e., something was done to look for cause of multiple cancers within the family	Extra surveillance unnecessary as cancer risk would be the same as for the general population
Reduction of uncertainty and anxiety	**Risks**	Relief that children cannot inherit the altered gene
Ability to test other family members for known mutation within the family	Anxiety and depression over uncertain results	Financial savings from decreased surveillance
Reason as to "why" cancer developed	Family continues to be monitored as a high-risk family	Decreased anxiety about ability to plan for the future
Risks	"No news"	Relief over not having greatly increased risk for developing cancer
Anxiety and depression over increased cancer risk	Current testing techniques and state of knowledge cannot classify all mutations as positive (deleterious) or negative	**Risks**
Fear that "nothing can be done" to minimize risk for developing cancer		Delay in seeking recommended cancer screening measures
Lowered life goals		Survivor guilt
Strained relationships within family (e.g., guilt over passing mutation to children)		Depression because increased cancer risks can no longer serve as cause of problems
Potential for discrimination by employers, insurers, and state licensing agencies		Strained relationships within the family
Financial costs of cancer screening and detection		
Positive tests predict risk of developing disease, not occurrence of cancer; age or time of developing cancer unknown		

*When there is a known mutation within the family

IV. Models for Cancer Risk Counseling Programs[41–43]

A. No standard model exists for a cancer risk evaluation program that specifically addresses the unique issues associated with genetic testing.

B. An effective program would include:

1. *Clinical and psychosocial assessment,*

2. *Education,*

3. *Individualized cancer risk analysis,*

4. *Genetic counseling, and*

5. *Long-term screening and surveillance for cancer (preferably within the context of a primary prevention program).*

C. In many institutions, centers providing cancer genetic counseling services are housed within prevention centers, as opposed to disease site centers. Cancer predisposition genes cause patterns of cancer that often do not respect current disease site center boundaries. Patients may also prefer to be seen in a "wellness" setting versus an "illness" setting, if they do not have a diagnosis of cancer.

D. A variety of healthcare professionals with specialized training currently provide cancer genetic counseling. These professionals include oncologists, oncology nurses with specialized training in cancer genetics, genetic counselors with specialized training in oncology, and medical geneticists.

E. Credentials that recognize expertise in the field of cancer genetic counseling or genetics are evolving for nurses. An initial attempt to recognize expertise in cancer genetics was initiated in May 2000. Offered by the Institute for Clinical Evaluation (I.C.E.), the credential was developed to attest to competence in Familial Cancer Risk Assessment and Management (FCRAM).

1. *The FCRAM credential was intended for advanced-practice nurses, physicians, genetic counselors, and other health care professionals who provide risk analysis and clinical cancer counseling service to patients who have or who are thought to be at risk for cancer.*

2. *The credentialing process assesses the knowledge and skills about clinical syndromes, clinical management, quantitative aspects/population genetics, basic science, and ethical/legal issues.*

3. *The first exam was administered in May 2001. Since then, the American Board of Internal Medicine (ABIM) Foundation has announced the phasing out of the I.C.E. credentialing program as an entity within the ABIM Foundation. The Foundation Trustees have appointed a transition team to explore the transfer of I.C.E. credentialing activities to another entity. The qualifications of those holding I.C.E. credentials will continue to be verified by the ABIM Foundation for the duration of a certificate's validity.*

4. *The International Society of Nurses in Genetics, a nursing specialty organization dedicated to fostering the scientific and professional growth of nurses in human genetics, has a credentialing committee that initiated a process for awarding*

a credential in genetics for advanced-practice nurses. As of May 2002, thirteen credentials for advanced-practice nurses in genetics have been awarded (www.isong.org).

V.   **Implications for Healthcare Providers**[44-53]

A.   All licensed healthcare providers, regardless of their practice setting, will have a role in the delivery of genetic services and the management of genetic information.

B.   Healthcare professionals will require genetic knowledge to identify, refer, support, and care for persons affected by or at risk for manifesting or transmitting genetic conditions.

C.   Assessment of family history as it relates to cancer will become increasingly important in cancer care whenever assessment of risk is performed for cancers such as breast cancer.

D.   See Table 11.5 for an overview of characteristics seen in families with a hereditary cancer syndrome.

E.   It is important to be aware of clinics that offer specialized cancer risk counseling services so that appropriate referrals can be made for patients with high-risk features or who are anxious about their family history.

References

1. International Society of Nurses in Genetics. *American Nurses Association: Statement on the Scope and Standards of Genetics Clinical Nursing Practice.* Washington, DC: American Nurses Publishing; 1998:1–42.

2. National Society of Genetic Counselors, Inc. *Genetic Counseling as a Profession.* Adopted 1994.: National Society of Genetic Counselors; Wallingford, PA. http://www.nsgc.org/CareerInformation. Accessed 9-2002.

3. Secretary's Advisory Committee on Genetic Testing Web site. Available at: http://www4.od.nih.gov/oba/sacgt/gtdocuments.html.

4. Rieger PT. Counseling on genetic risk for cancer. In: Yarbro CH, Hansen Frogge M, Goodman M, Groenwald SL, eds. *Cancer Nursing: Principles and Practice.* 5th ed. Sudbury, MA: Jones and Bartlett Publishers; 2000:189–213.

5. Cummings S. The genetic testing process: how much counseling is needed? *J Clin Oncol* 2000;18(suppl 21):60S–64S.

6. Cummings S, Olopade OI. Predisposition testing for breast cancer. *Oncol* 1998;12:1227–1242.

7. Lea D, Jenkins JF, Francomano C. *Genetics in Clinical Practice: New Directions for Nursing and Health Care.* Boston, MA: Jones & Bartlett Publishers; 1998:1–262.

8. Peters JA, Stopfer JE. Role of the genetic counselor in familial cancer risk. *Oncol* 1996;10:159–175.

9. Rieger PT. Overview of cancer and genetics: implications for nurse practitioners. *Nurs Pract Forum* 1998;9:122–133.

10. Schneider KA. *Counseling about Cancer.* 2nd ed. New York, NY: Wiley; 2001.

11. Stopfer JE. Genetic counseling and clinical cancer genetics services. *Semin Surg Oncol* June 2000;18:347–357.

12. Offit K. *Clinical Cancer Genetics: Risk Counseling and Management.* New York, NY: Wiley-Liss; 1998:1–448.

13. Bennett RL. *The Practical Guide to Genetic Family History.* New York, NY: Wiley-Liss; 1999:1–251.

14. Loescher LJ. The family history component of cancer genetic risk counseling. *Cancer Nurs* 1999;22:96–102.

15. Mahon SM. Cancer risk assessment: conceptual considerations for clinical practice. *Oncol Nurs Forum* 1998;25:1535–1547.

16. Iglehart JD, Miron A, Rimer BK, et al. Overestimation of hereditary breast cancer risk. *Ann Surg* 1998;228:375–384.

17. Vogel V. Assessing women's potential risk of developing breast cancer. *Oncol* 1996;10:1451–1458, 1461; discussion 1462–1463.

18. Lindor NM, Greene MH. The concise handbook of family cancer syndromes. Mayo Familial Cancer Program. *J Natl Cancer Inst* 1998;90:1039–1071.

19. Burke W, Daly M, Garber JE, et al. Recommendations for follow-up care of individuals with an inherited predisposition to cancer. II. BRCA1 and BRCA2. *JAMA* 1997;277:997–1003.

20. Daly M. NCCN practice guidelines: genetics/familial high-risk cancer screening. *Oncol* 1999;13:161–183.

21. NCCN. *NCCN Guidelines: Genetics/Familial High-Risk Cancer Screening* [book on CD-ROM]. Rockledge, Pa:NCCN; 2001. Based on: *The Complete Library of NCCN Oncology Practice Guidelines.*

22. King MC, Wieand S, Hale K, et al. National Surgical Adjuvant Breast and Bowel Project. Tamoxifen and breast cancer incidence among women with inherited mutations in BRCA1 and BRCA2: National Surgical Adjuvant Breast and Bowel Project (NSABP–P1) Breast Cancer Prevention Trial. *JAMA* 2001;286:2251–2256.

23. Modan B, Hartge P, Hirsh-Yechezkel G, et al. National Israel Ovarian Cancer Study Group. Parity, oral contraceptives, and the risk of ovarian cancer among carriers and noncarriers of a BRCA1 or BRCA2 mutation. *N Engl J Med* 2001;345:235–240.

24. Narod SA, Boyd J. Current understanding of the epidemiology and clinical implications of BRCA1 and BRCA2 mutations for ovarian cancer. *Curr Opin Obstet Gynecol* 2002;14:19–26.

25. Hartmann LC, Schaid DJ, Woods JE, et al. Efficacy of bilateral prophylactic mastectomy in women with a family history of breast cancer. *N Engl J Med* 1999;340:77–84.

26. Hartmann LC, Sellers TA, Schaid DJ, et al. Efficacy of bilateral prophylactic mastectomy in BRCA1 and BRCA2 gene mutation carriers. *J Natl Cancer Inst* 2001;93:1633–1637.

27. Meijers-Heijboer H, van Geel B, van Putten WL, et al. Breast cancer after prophylactic bilateral mastectomy in women with a BRCA1 or BRCA2 mutation. *N Engl J Med* 2001;345:159–164.

28. Kauff ND, Satagopan JM, Robson ME., et al. Risk-reducing salpingo-oophorectomy in women with a BRCA1 or BRCA2 mutation. *N Engl J Med* 2002;346:1609–1615.

29. Bove C, Fry ST, MacDonald DJ. Presymptomatic and predisposition genetic testing: ethical and social considerations. *Sem Oncol Nurs* 1997;13:135–140.

30. Jacobs LA. At-Risk for cancer: genetic discrimination in the workplace. *Oncol Nurs Forum* 1998;25:475–480.

31. Tercyak KP, Lerman C, Peshkin BN, et al. Effects of coping style and BRCA1 and BRCA2 test results on anxiety among women participating in genetic counseling and testing for breast and ovarian cancer risk. *Health Psychol* 2001;20:217–222.

32. Daly MB, Barsevick A, Miller SM, et al. Communicating genetic test results to the family: a six-step, skills-building strategy. *Fam Community Health* 2001;24:13–26.

33. Di Prospero LS, Seminsky M, Honeyford J, et al. Psychosocial issues following a positive result of genetic testing for BRCA1 and BRCA2 mutations: findings from a focus group and a needs-assessment survey. *CMAJ* 2001;164:1005–1009.

34. Lerman C, Croyle RT. Emotional and behavioral responses to genetic testing for susceptibility to cancer. *Oncol* 1996;10:191–199.

35. American Society of Clinical Oncology. Statement of the American Society of Clinical Oncology: genetic testing for cancer susceptibility. *J Clin Oncol* 1996;14:1730–1736.

36. American Society of Human Genetics. Genetic testing for breast and ovarian cancer predisposition. *Am J Hum Genet* 1994;55:i–iv.

37. Geller G, Botkin JR, Green MJ, et al. Genetic testing for susceptibility to adult-onset cancer: the process and content of informed consent. *JAMA* 1997;277:1471–1474.

38. Rieger PT, Pentz RB. Genetic testing and informed consent. *Semin Oncol Nurs* 1999;2:104–115.

39. Peshkin BN, DeMarco TA, Brogan BM, et al. BRCA1/2 testing: complex themes in result interpretation. *J Clin Oncol* 2001;19:2555–2565.

40. Lawrence WF, Peshkin BN, Liang W, et al. Cost of genetic counseling and testing for BRCA1 and BRCA2 breast cancer susceptibility mutations. *Cancer Epidemiol Biomarkers Prev* 2001;10:475–481.

41. Calzone KA, Stopfer J, Blackwood A, Weber BL. Establishing a cancer risk evaluation program. *Cancer Pract* 1997;5:228–233.

42. Mills GB, Rieger PT. Genetic predisposition to breast cancer. In: Hunt KK, Robb GL, Strom EA, Ueno N. *Breast Cancer*. New York, NY: Springer-Verlag; 2001:55–92.

43. Pichert G, Stahel RA. Organizing cancer genetics programs: the Swiss model. *J Clin Oncol* 2000;18(suppl 21):65S–69S.

44. Olopade OI, Pichert G. Cancer genetics in oncology practice. *Ann Oncol* 2001;12:895–908.

45. Calzone KA. Genetic predisposition testing: clinical implications for oncology nurses. *Oncol Nurs Forum* 1997;24:712–718.

46. Collins FS, Jenkins JF. Implications of the human genome project for the nursing profession. In: Lashley FR. *The Genetic Revolution: Implications for Nursing*. Washington, DC: American Academy of Nursing; 1997:9–13.

47. Dimond E, Calzone KA, Davis J, Jenkins JF. The role of the nurse in cancer genetics. *Can Nurs* 1998;21:57–75.

48. Emery J, Lucassen A, Murphy M. Common hereditary cancers and implications for primary care. *Lancet* 2001;358:56–63.

49. Johnson KA, Brensinger JD. Genetic counseling and testing: implications for clinical practice. *Nurs Clin North Am* 2000;35:615–626.

50. MacDonald DJ. The oncology nurse's role in cancer risk assessment and counseling. *Semin Oncol Nursing* 1997;13:123–128.

51. National Center for Human Genome Research. *The Human Genome Project: From maps to medicine*. Bethesda, Md: Department of Health and Human Services Public Health Service; 1995. NIH Publication 96–3897.

52. Oncology Nursing Society. ONS position statement: cancer predisposition genetic testing and risk assessment counseling. *Oncol Nurs Forum* 2000;27:1349.

53. Oncology Nursing Society. ONS position statement: the role of the oncology nurse in cancer genetic counseling. *Oncol Nurs Forum* 2000;27:1348.

chapter 12

Psychological Management of Women at Increased Risk

Susan R. Stollings, PhD
Senior Clinician, Behavioral Medicine and Oncology
University of Pittsburgh Cancer Institute
Pittsburgh, PA

I. **Definition, Characteristics, and Function of Worry**
A. Definition of Worry: "Worry is a chain of thoughts and images, negatively affect laden and relatively uncontrollable; it represents an attempt to engage in mental problem-solving on an issue whose outcome is uncertain but contains the possibility of one or more negative outcomes."[1]
B. Characteristics of Worry.[1,2,3]
1. *Future oriented—usually about what "might" happen in the future*
2. *Primarily a cognitive process*
3. *"Self-perpetuating"—may result in somatic symptoms that are misinterpreted as serious, thereby resulting in further increases in worry*
4. *Correlates with fear, anxiety, and depression*
5. *Leads to interpretation of ambiguous or uncertain information as threatening*
6. *Feelings of vulnerability and powerlessness for the worried individual*
7. *Often involves use of suboptimal coping (e.g., avoidance) and/or lack of adaptive problem-solving or coping skills*
C. Functions of Worry.[1,4]
1. *Negative aspects of worry*
a. The individual has a superstitious belief that negative outcomes can be avoided or prevented through worry.
b. Worry serves as distraction from or avoidance of other issues, for example, patient may use worry about health to avoid facing marital difficulties.
c. Worry also serves as preparation for coping with a feared outcome, that is, if one is prepared for the worst case scenario, one will be able to cope with it. This may be maladaptive because the focus is on negative outcomes that are largely unlikely to occur.
2. *Positive aspects of worry*
a. Motivational function—If the patient is worried about a breast lump, worry may motivate the patient to get a mammogram.
b. "Wake-up call"—Worry may highlight or focus attention on salient issues, such as getting one's priorities in order.

II. **Cancer-Related Worry—General Issues and Issues Pregenetic Counseling**
A. Cancer is one of the most feared illnesses among patients with health anxiety.[5,6]
B. One study of 1,012 women ages 30 to 49 in a primary care setting indicated that 48% of respondents rated their degree of worry about being diagnosed with breast cancer as moderate or very worried.[7]
C. Only 30 to 40% of patients correctly estimate their personal risk for breast cancer, often because of lack of knowledge of cancer risk factors and rates. Misperceptions about risk may be difficult to correct.[8]

FIGURE 12.1	Factors Affecting Cancer Worry or Anxiety

	Perceived likelihood of illness	$\times$	Perceived cost, awfulness and burden of the illness
Anxiety =			
	Perceived ability to cope with the illness	$+$	Perception of the extent to which external factors will help (rescue factors)

From *Hypochondriasis* by Vladan Starcevic and Don Lipsitt, copyright 2001 by Oxford University Press, Inc. Used by permission of Oxford University Press, Inc.

D. Women who have mammographic abnormalities and/or false-positive mammographic results appear to have significantly greater worry than women with normal results.[9]

E. Younger women appear to report greater distress than older women.[8]

F. Single women appear to report greater distress than married women.[10]

G. African-American women reported greater distress about cancer risk than Caucasian women in a study of 256 women who requested genetic counseling/testing.[10]

H. Worry may be based on a patient's perceptions of cancer and its ramifications (see Figure 12.1).[11]

I. Worry may have a curvilinear relationship to screening, in that too much worry or not enough worry may result in lack of patient adherence to recommended cancer screening, while a moderate amount of worry may motivate screening behavior.[8,9]

J. Worry may increase at the age when a first-degree relative (FDR) developed cancer.[12]

K. Women may lack social support because they do not want to "burden" friends or family or if they perceive that friends or family do not understand why they are worried.[12]

L. Uncertainty contributes to worry and may motivate a person to pursue genetic counseling or testing.[9]

M. Patients at high risk for cancer often report shame or anger about being at elevated risk.[9]

N. Women with an optimistic outlook appear to worry less and report less distress than women with a pessimistic outlook who may have greater difficulty coping with genetic test results.[10]

O. Perceived control over one's health was found to be negatively correlated with worry about cancer risk, particularly when risk was felt to be low.[10]

P. Individuals with low self-esteem often have higher health anxiety than individuals with high self-esteem.[11]

Q. Worried individuals tend to be particularly attentive to cancer-related information and have increased focus on bodily symptoms.[13]

III.   **Worry in Women Who Have Been Tested for BRCA1 and BRAC2**
   A. Negative Results
      1. *Usually results in feeling of relief*[14,15]
      2. *May also result in numbness or "survivor's guilt"*[15]
      3. *May not be alleviated as a negative finding may not completely reduce a patient's risk*[16]
   B. Positive Results
      1. *A positive result usually results in more distress than a negative result.*
      2. *Distress may be greater if patients have no family history of cancer or no personal history of breast surgery,*[17] *either because they were not expecting a positive result and/or because they may feel that they have not developed coping skills applicable to this stressor.*
      3. *Worry is increased if patients feel there is no manner in which to cope with test results or protect themselves from cancer in the future.*[16]
   C. General Issues
      1. *Emotional reaction may depend on premorbid personality issues.*
         a. Patients high on monitoring (seeking and focusing on health issues) may have more distress than patients high on blunting (downplaying or avoiding health information).[8,14]
         b. Patients who were more worried before testing and/or had intrusive thoughts are likely to be more worried and/or have intrusive thoughts after testing compared to patients in general.[15]
         c. Depressed individuals may notice greater worry or distress after testing.[15]
         d. Patients who are pessimistic are likely to be more distressed and/or avoid appropriate surveillance.[8]
         e. Neuroticism is associated with greater distress.[8]
         f. Social support is negatively correlated with distress.[8]
      2. *Waiting for results is a particularly stressful situation.*[14]
      3. *Distress appears to decrease after results are disclosed regardless of findings,*[15,17] *perhaps because of a reduction in uncertainty.*[9]
      4. *DudokdeWit and colleagues found that individuals with children had increased distress regardless of genetic test result because of lingering concerns of having passed a disease on to one's children.*[15]
      5. *Individuals who refuse genetic testing may be at risk for increased worry, distress, or depression that may inhibit appropriate cancer screening. It is recommended that these individuals be followed carefully for signs of stress.*[18]

IV.   **When to Refer Worried Patients for Psychological Intervention**
   A. Behavioral Indicators of Excessive Worry
      1. *Excessive Breast Self Examination (BSE). One study of first-degree relatives of patients with breast cancer indicated 8% of 1,053 subjects performed BSE daily or more often.*

Characteristics associated with excessive BSE included older age, lesser education, race (African-American), having a daughter, and/or two or more FDRs with breast cancer.[6]

2. *Other excessive health behaviors, including seeking multiple and/or unnecessary medical tests, examinations, procedures, or opinions.*[11]

3. *Making multiple telephone calls to medical team for reassurance.*

4. *Consistently misinterpreting benign symptoms as signs of a serious illness.*[11]

5. *Avoiding recommended screening and/or diagnostic tests and procedures, which artificially relieves worry based on the superstitious belief that cancer cannot be discovered if one is not tested for it.*[8]

6. *Sleep disturbance individual being unable to fall asleep or stay asleep.*

7. *Significant changes in eating patterns.*

8. *Avoidance of family or friends and/or avoidance of pleasurable social activities.*

9. *Impaired work at job or home compared to usual levels.*

10. *Motor agitation.*

11. *Excessive tearfulness.*

12. *Increased used of alcohol, tobacco, prescription, or nonprescription drugs.*[8]

B. Psychological/Emotional Indicators of Excessive Worry— particularly those that result in difficulties socially or professionally or that impair quality of life

1. *Extended periods of sad or irritable mood*

2. *Extended periods of anxiety*

3. *Racing thoughts*

4. *Ruminating on health with inability to shift thinking to more neutral topics*

5. *Intrusive thoughts of an upsetting nature*

6. *Inability to be reassured by family, friends, or medical team*

7. *Thoughts of death manifested as:*
   a. Fear of dying
   b. Sadness or distress about family's likely reactions to one's death
   c. Obsessive thoughts about "getting affairs in order" to the exclusion of other thoughts despite having a low risk of cancer
   d. Suicidal ideation

C. Other Indications for Referral

1. *Physician feels he or she is unable to work productively with patient.*[19]

2. *Patient feels unable to work productively with physician.*

D. General Categories of Psychological Diagnoses That May Cause or Explain Excessive Worry in Patients at High Risk for Developing Breast Cancer[11,20]

1. *Anxiety disorders.*
    a. Generalized Anxiety Disorder (GAD)—This disorder is manifested as worry about a variety of topics that occurs more often than not for six months or more. Many patients report anxiety beginning in childhood. The lifetime prevalence is 5%. Approximately 55 to 60% of individuals with GAD are women.
    b. Specific Phobia—In the health setting, this disorder may be manifested as fear of death, fear of illness, or fear of blood, injection, or injury. The lifetime prevalence of this disorder is 10 to 11.3%, and 55 to 70% of individuals with this disorder are women.
    c. Panic Disorder—The main symptom of this disorder is panic attacks that are perpetuated by worry about future panic attacks. The lifetime prevalence of panic disorder is 1.5 to 3.0%. It often occurs between adolescence and mid-thirties and is more prevalent in women.
    d. Obsessive-Compulsive Disorder (OCD)—OCD may involve obsessive thoughts about illness and/or compulsive behaviors such as excessive BSE or physician consultations. The lifetime prevalence is 2.5%. It is equally likely to occur in men and women.

2. *Depressive Disorder—Depression is often associated with preoccupation with and/or excessive focus on negative aspects of situations. Individuals at high risk for breast cancer who are depressed may become convinced that they will definitely develop breast cancer and that they will be unable to cope with it, while negating evidence to the contrary. They are also more likely to notice somatic complaints such as pain. Depressive symptoms must be present for at least two weeks to meet DSM-IV criteria for diagnosis. Depression is roughly twice as prevalent in women as men.*

3. *Somatoform Disorders—This class of disorders applies to "physical symptoms that suggest a general medical condition . . . and are not fully explained by a general medical condition, by the direct effects of a substance, or by another mental disorder."[20, p. 445] Subtypes include:*
    a. Somatization Disorder—The hallmark of this disorder is that the patient reports complaints of pain or physical symptoms in at least four separate body systems in the absence of or over and above medically justified conditions. Somatization usually begins before age 30 and is more prevalent in women (lifetime prevalence in females is 0.2 to 2%).
    b. Hypochondriasis—The prominent symptom is excessive worry that one has or might have a medical disorder despite reassurance or evidence to the contrary. This disorder is found equally in men and women.
    c. Body Dysmorphic Disorder—Individuals with this disorder evidence a "preoccupation with a defect in appearance . . . either imagined or, if a slight physical anomaly is present, the individual's concern is markedly excessive."[20, p. 466] It occurs equally in females and males.

4. *Other.*
    a. Psychosis—The patient may have a delusional belief that he or she has or will develop cancer.
    b. Personality Disorder—Worry about cancer may result in secondary gain (e.g., attention).

V.   **Interventions for Worried Patients**

   A.   What Patients Can Do on Their Own to Cope with Worries about Cancer[2,4]

   1.   *Focus on health behaviors they can control, such as healthier eating habits, exercise, quitting smoking, and so forth.*

   2.   *Maintain a focus on the present rather than the future.*

   3.   *Use distraction techniques, for example, if one is bothered by intrusive thoughts about cancer, engage interest in a diverting activity such as reading, viewing a movie, and the like.*

   4.   *Use meditation and relaxation techniques.*

   5.   *Utilize active problem-solving to cope with problems that are "solvable," for example, if a patient does not understand a test result, the patient calls the physician for an explanation rather than avoiding calling, which would increase worry.*

   6.   *Use positive self-talk. The patient can develop personal coping statements (such as "I am exercising to stay healthy and following my treatment plan") and repeat them to himself or herself during times of worry.*

   7.   *Ask the patient to keep a journal, which may help to work through anxiety. Research on keeping a journal indicates that regularly writing about a traumatic subject may be related to improved health and outlook.[21]*

   B.   Interventions That Can Be Done by the Medical Team

   1.   *Institute reminders about screening including personalized risk information via telephone or mail.[8]*

   2.   *Reduce the amount of time that patients wait for test results.[8]*

   3.   *Educate the patient about actual risk for cancer when the patient is overestimating or underestimating risk.[8]*

   4.   *Remind patients of information that was discussed, as anxiety may interfere with patients' ability to concentrate or remember the information.[8]*

   5.   *Teach patients easy relaxation techniques such as diaphragmatic breathing.[12]*

   6.   *Support patients' positive health behaviors and offer suggestions to maximize use of prevention strategies.[11]*

   7.   *Work collaboratively with patients to establish guidelines on screening that are mutually acceptable.*

   8.   *The physician should present a calm demeanor and be respectful of the patient, being alert to other stressors that may be exacerbating patient's worry.[22]*

   C.   Psychological/Psychiatric Interventions

   1.   *Cognitive-Behavioral Therapy—This form of therapy is based on the theory that patient's thought patterns contain distortions that result in anxiety or depression. Once these distortions are corrected, psychological symptoms abate. This therapy has been studied with patients diagnosed with hypochondriasis and was superior to a control group of patients on a waiting list.[3,13,23,24] It includes the following techniques:*

   a.   Psychoeducation regarding the relationship between thoughts and emotions.

   b. Identification of distorted thoughts (e.g., My chance of developing cancer is 100%).
   c. Education about challenging these thoughts through examination of evidence or through behavioral experiments (e.g., If the patient states he or she has never met anyone who lived for more than one year after a cancer diagnosis, help the patient identify individuals who have lived more than one year after cancer diagnosis).
   d. Encouragement of continued examination of thoughts through homework assignments.
   e. Individualized treatment to target the patient's specific thoughts.
   f. Apparent continuation of treatment gains at least 3 to 12 months after treatment has ended.
   g. Achievement of a sense of control for patients as an important treatment goal.

2. *Behavioral Therapy—This therapy was also found to be superior to no intervention in clinical studies. It may be less effective in the short term than cognitive behavioral therapy but appears to be as effective at follow-up.*[13,24]
   a. This therapy involves psychoeducation about anxiety/worry and use of relaxation techniques, problem-solving strategies, assertive communication, and the role of avoidance in perpetuating anxiety.
   b. The therapist works with the patient on developing a hierarchy of fears, working up from least feared situation to most feared situation.
   c. The therapist also works with the patient and family to extinguish avoidance behaviors or help patients confront feared situations such as having a mammogram that the patient may have avoided before therapy.
   d. A specified "worry time" is assigned each day to decrease the overall amount of time spent worrying.

3. *Group Interventions—There is limited research in this area, but one study found that a six-week psychoeducational group was more effective in increasing breast cancer risk knowledge and breast cancer screening than a control group.*[25]

4. *Explanatory Therapy*[26]*—This therapy was developed for use in patients with hypochondriasis.*
   a. It involves reattributing body symptoms as benign and providing "accurate information" to patients. There is also a component of support. Repetition is a key factor in assisting with information retention.
   b. The benefits of this therapy are that it is atheoretical and can be provided by trained paraprofessionals.
   c. The treatment protocol involves meeting every other week for 16 weeks.
   d. A study of 20 patients found that explanatory therapy was superior to wait list in decreasing distress and decreasing medical visits.
   e. Treatment gains were evident at 6-month follow-up.

5. *Psychopharmacology (based on personal communication with Malhotra S. October 16, 2001).*
   a. Medications for acute anxiety—First line treatment is use of benzodiazepines.
   b. Medications for chronic anxiety.

    i.   Approval of most selective serotonin reuptake inhibitors for treating anxiety

    ii.   Serotonin agonists (e.g., Buspirone hydrochloride)

    iii.   Second-generation antidepressants such as Mirtazapine, Nefazodone, Venlafaxine, and Buproprion HCl

    iv.   Tricyclic antidepressants

References

1. Borkovec TE. The nature, function, and origin of worry. In: Davey GCL, Tallis F, eds. *Worrying: Perspectives on Theory, Assessment, and Treatment.* New York, NY: John Wiley and Sons; 1994:7.

2. Hallowell EM. *Worry: Controlling It and Using It Wisely.* New York, NY: Pantheon; 1997.

3. Hadjistavropoulos HD, Craig KD, Hadjistavropoulos T. Cognitive and behavioral responses to illness information: the role of health anxiety. *Behav Res and Ther* 1998;36:149–164.

4. Copeland ME. *The Worry Control Workbook.* Oakland, CA: New Harbinger; 1998.

5. Barsky AJ, Ahern DK, Baily ED, Saintfort R, Liu EB, Peekna HM. Hypochondriacal patients' appraisal of health and physical risks. *Am J Psychiatry* 2001;158:783–787.

6. Epstein SA, Lerman C. Excessive health behaviors in those at risk for physical disorder. *J Psychosomatic Res* 1997;43:223–225.

7. Kinsinger L, Harris R, Karnitschnig J. Worry about breast cancer in younger women: a major problem. *J Gen Intern Med* 1998;13(suppl 1):99.

8. Posluszny DM, Baum A. Psychological management of women at risk for breast cancer. In: Vogel VG, ed. *Management of Patients at High Risk for Breast Cancer.* Malden, MA: Blackwell Science Inc; 2001:228–244.

9. Croyle RT, ed. *Psychosocial Effects of Screening for Disease Prevention and Detection.* New York, NY: Oxford University Press; 1995.

10. Audrain J, Schwartz MD, Lerman C, Hughes C, Peshkin BN, Biesecker B. Psychological distress in women seeking genetic counseling for breast-ovarian cancer risk: the contributions of personality and appraisal. *Ann Behav Med* 1998;19:370–377.

11. Starcevic V, Lipsitt DR, eds. *Hypochondriasis: Modern Perspectives on an Ancient Malady.* New York, NY: Oxford University Press; 2001.

12. Kash KM, Lerman C. Psychological, social, and ethical issues in gene testing. In: Holland JC, ed. *Psycho-oncology.* New York, NY: Oxford University Press; 1998:196–207.

13. Warwick HMC, Clark DM, Cobb AM, Salkovskis PM. A controlled trial of cognitive-behavioural treatment of hypochondriasis. *Br J Psychiatry* 1996;169:189–195.

14. Tercyak KP, Lerman C, Peshkin BN, et al. Aspects of coping style and BRCA1 and BRCA2 test results on anxiety among women participating in genetic counseling and testing for breast and ovarian cancer risk. *Health Psychol* 2001;20:217–222.

15. DudokdeWit AC, Tibben A, Duivenvoorden HJ, Niermeijer MF, Passchier J. Predicting adaptation to presymptomatic DNA testing for late onset disorders: who will experience distress? *J Med Genet* 1998;35:745–754.

16. Lerman C. Psychological aspects of genetic testing for cancer susceptibility. In: Krantz DS, Baum A, eds. *Technology and Methods in Behavioral Medicine.* Mahwah, NJ: Lawrence Erlbaum Associates; 1998:15–28.

17. Croyle RT, Smith KR, Botkin JR, Baty B, Nash J. Psychological responses to BRCA1 mutation testing: preliminary findings. *Health Psychol* 1997;16:63–72.

18. Lerman C, Hughes C, Lemon SJ, et al. What you don't know can hurt you: adverse psychologic effects in members of BRCA1-linked and BRCA2-linked families who decline genetic testing. *J Clin Oncol* 1998;16:1650–1654.

19. Beckman HB. Difficult patients. In: Feldman MD, Christensen JF, eds. *Behavioral Medicine in Primary Care: a Practical Guide.* Stamford, CT: Appleton & Lange; 1997:20–29.

20. American Psychiatric Association. *Diagnostic and Statistical Manual of Mental Disorders.* 4th ed. Washington, DC: American Psychiatric Association; 1994.

21. Pennebaker JW. Emotion, disclosure, and health: an overview. In: Pennebaker JW, ed. *Emotion, Disclosure, and Health.* Washington, DC: American Psychological Association; 1995;3–8.

22. Blackwell B, DeMorgan NP. The primary care of patients who have bodily concerns. *Arch Fam Med* 1996;5:457–463.

23. Visser S, Bouman TK. The treatment of hypochondriasis: exposure plus response prevention vs. cognitive therapy. *Behav Res and Therapy* 2001;39:423–442.

24. Clark DM, Salkovskis PM, Hackmann A, et al. Two psychological treatments for hypochondriasis. a randomised controlled trial. *Br J Psychiatry* 1998;173:218–225.

25. Schwartz MD, Lerman C, Rimer B. Psychosocial interventions for women at increased risk for breast cancer. In: Baum A, Andersen BL, eds. *Psychosocial Interventions for Cancer.* Washington, DC: American Psychological Association; 2001:287–304.

26. Fava GA, Grandi S, Rafanelli C, Fabbri S, Cazzaro M. Explanatory therapy in hypochondriasis. *J Clin Psychiatry* 2000;61:317–322.

chapter 13

Cost Effectiveness of Breast Cancer Risk Management

Suzanne Day, MSN, RN, CS, FNP
Family Nurse Practitioner
Cancer Prevention Center
The University of Texas M.D. Anderson Cancer Center
Houston, TX

I.   **Introduction**

   A. Technology makes breast cancer screening possible. There is a
       lack of consensus, however, between advisory groups as to the
       optimal age to begin screening and the most cost-effective
       interval between screenings. Routine screening
       recommendations may be inadequate for individuals at
       increased risk for breast cancer, and several advisory groups
       have recommended more intensive screening for these
       individuals.

   B. With limited healthcare funds, careful selection of individuals
       at increased risk for breast cancer is necessary to assure
       appropriate allocation of resources. Individuals not found to be
       at increased risk can be followed with less costly routine
       screening recommendations.

   C. The selection of high to moderate risk women and counseling
       them regarding their options is a complex and time-intensive
       process. Midlevel providers, as members of a multidisciplinary
       team, may be particularly well suited to this task. Nurse
       practitioners have been found to provide care that is well
       accepted by patients and is cost effective even with slightly
       longer clinic visits.[1,2]

II. **Screening for Genetic Risk of Breast Cancer**

   A. Demand for testing

       1. *The identification and development of a commercially
           marketed test for Breast Cancer 1 (BRCA1) and Breast Cancer 2
           (BRCA2) genes has created a demand for this testing.*

       2. *Women with significant family history may wish to confirm
           their perception of significant risk for breast cancer.*

       3. *Healthcare providers may suggest genetic testing to clarify an
           individual's risk for breast cancer in order to plan the most
           effective care.*

   B. Cost effectiveness of positive test for BRCA1 or BRCA2

       1. *The outcome of this testing has significant implications for the
           management of high-risk individuals.*

           a. While genetic testing may involve a significant initial cost
               (Table 13.1), individuals who test negative may have to be
               moved out of an intensive screening schedule (Table 13.2)
               into a less costly screening follow-up. In addition,
               prophylactic surgery can be avoided.

           b. Conversely, individuals who test positive for BRCA1 or BRCA2
               can be targeted for intensive screening and prevention
               strategies (Table 13.2). Cost effectiveness of positive genetic
               testing varies significantly with the woman's course of
               treatment. In women of Ashkenazi Jewish descent, genetic
               testing has been demonstrated to be cost effective when
               followed with prophylactic surgery.[3]

       2. *Counseling for genetic testing.*

           a. The cost of counseling must be included in any evaluation of
               cost effectiveness. Genetic testing requires that significant
               time be spent counseling prior to testing and following
               receipt of results. According to personal communication
               with P. Rieger in August 2001, the fee for counseling has been

TABLE 13.1	Cost of BRCA1 and BRCA2 Testing	
BRCA Test	Cost per Test	Other Charges to Consider
Comprehensive testing for BRCA1 and BRCA2	$2,760	Cost for counseling ($300 to > $750)
Limited testing of three common mutations among individuals of Ashkenazi Jewish descent	$385	Cost of counseling ($300 to > $750); Additional testing of other mutations if three common sites are negative ($2,450)
Testing of single mutation with known family mutation	$325	Testing and counseling of index case relative to identify mutation; Cost of counseling ($300 to > $750); Will not identify second mutation present in rare cases

For additional information or current prices, contact Myriad Genetic Laboratories, Inc., 320 Wakara Way, Salt Lake City, UT 84108, 1-800-725-2722.

        estimated to add anywhere from approximately $300[3] to over $750 to the cost of testing. Note that the costs quoted in Table 13.1 are the cost of testing and do not include counseling.

   b. The initial review of the family history is an integral part of genetic testing; however, to limit costs while assuring accuracy, this step can be performed by clinic staff prior to scheduling a counseling appointment. This review serves to reduce costly counseling of inappropriate families, such as very small families and families with insufficient data to support testing.

   c. The family practice physician may have neither the time nor the expertise to adequately counsel the individual. The midlevel provider functioning in a specialty clinic may be a more appropriate choice for counseling in terms of both cost and expertise. For example, a nurse practitioner of national reputation is a critical member of the team that offers family risk assessment in a comprehensive cancer center. Extensive education and experience enables this nurse practitioner to provide a desired service within a marketable cost.

3. *Cost to test for BRCA1 and BRCA2.*

   a. Test costs vary widely depending on the background of the individual being tested (Table 13.1).

   b. The cost of a comprehensive BRCA1 and BRCA2 gene sequence analysis in an individual not of Ashkenazi Jewish decent and with no known family mutations would be $2,760. While this test identifies mutations in both the BRCA1 and BRCA2 genes, it does not identify unusual mutations or mutations that occur in unusual regions within the BRCA1 and BRCA2 genes.

   c. In women of Ashkenazi Jewish descent, a more limited test of the three most common BRCA1 and BRCA2 mutations found among this population can be performed at a cost of $385. However, if testing for these three mutations

TABLE 13.2	NCCN Screening Guidelines for Asymptotic Women at Increased Risk of Breast Cancer Age 25 or Older
Risk Category	**Screening Recommendations**
Strong family history or genetic predisposition	Annual mammogram and physical exam every 6 months starting at age 25 if BRCA positive and 5 to 10 years prior to age at diagnosis of youngest family member for women with strong family history; breast self-exam encouraged.
Prior radiation to chest wall	Annual mammogram and physical exam every 6 months starting 10 years following radiation; breast self-exam encouraged.
LCIS	Annual mammogram and physical exam every 6 to 12 months; breast self-exam encouraged.
Elevated risk for breast cancer > 1.67% in five years in women ≥ 35	Annual mammogram and annual physical exam; breast self-exam encouraged.

      is negative, additional testing for other potential mutations can be performed at a cost of $2,450.

d. If there is a known mutation within a family, a single site analysis can be offered to family members at a cost of $325. While the affected relative may require comprehensive BRCA1 and BRCA2 gene sequence analysis to identify a mutation, subsequent testing within that family may be limited to the less expensive single site analysis. A negative test would rule out only the known mutation but would not identify a second mutation in those rare families with multiple mutations. Comprehensive testing following a negative single site analysis would increase cost significantly.

e. In addition to the cost savings associated with a negative test, there are intangible benefits associated with a negative test, including reduced anxiety and less time spent in additional health screening and treatment.

III. **Use of the Modified Gail Model Risk Assessment Tool**

    A. This statistical model is used to estimate breast cancer risk. The model enables healthcare providers to identify women at increased risk for breast cancer. A woman with a five-year calculated risk of greater than or equal to 1.67% is considered to be at increased risk and may be a candidate for chemoprevention (see Section IX).

    B. Limitations of Modified Gail Model Risk Assessment.

        1. *The model has been well tested in Caucasian women but may be of less value in other racial/ethnic groups.*

        2. *It is not for use in women younger than age 35 or older than age 85.*

        3. *Only first-degree relatives are considered in this model.*

        4. *The age at diagnosis is not used in the calculation, and the model may therefore underestimate risk in women with a family history of early-onset breast cancers and may overestimate risk in women with elderly relatives diagnosed with breast cancer.*

        5. *The model does not predict risk for breast cancer among women with BRCA1 or BRCA2 mutations. Women with a strong family history of breast cancer or a family history of early-onset breast cancers may require genetic screening for a true appraisal of their risk (see Section V).*

    C. Cost to use Modified Gail Model Risk Assessment tool.

        1. *The computer program to calculate risk is available at no cost from the National Cancer Institute at http://bcra.nci.nih.gov/brc.*

        2. *The amount of time to collect necessary data to calculate risk is minimal and can be performed by office staff. Given the limitations of the model (see preceding) and the complexity of prevention options (see Section IX), significant time may be required from a knowledgeable individual to interpret results and discuss chemoprevention options. The cost effectiveness of this counseling would vary with the risk level of the population, the amount of time spent with individuals, and the number of individuals who elect chemoprevention. A follow-up office visit is often necessary to review risks and benefits of chemoprevention for those women who express an interest.*

IV. **Other Special Risk Factors for Breast Cancer**

    A. Lobular Carcinoma *In Situ* (LCIS)

        1. *The presence of LCIS increases risk of breast cancer by 4.2 to 9.3% in less than 5 years (overall incidence of 5.2%) and between 7.7 and 26.3% when followed for more than 5 years. The overall incidence of breast cancer is estimated to be 22.3%.*[4]

        2. *There are no additional costs associated with identification of women with LCIS. LCIS is an incidental finding noted during the evaluation process for other breast abnormalities.*

        3. *Risk reduction options.*

   a. Prophylactic mastectomy reduces risk by 90%.
   b. Chemoprevention with tamoxifen reduces risk by 56%.[5]
   c. These individuals may also elect to have increased surveillance (Table 13.2).

B. Atypical Ductal Hyperplasia (ADH)

   1. *The presence of ADH places a woman at 2.5 to 5.3 times the risk of breast cancer when compared to a woman without proliferative breast disease. ADH increases the risk of breast cancer 3.7 to 19.3% in less than 5 years (overall incidence of 6.4%, and between 13.6 to 33.6% when followed for more than 5 years. The overall incidence of breast cancer is estimated to be 19.5%.[4]*

   2. *Cost associated with diagnosis of ADH.*
      a. ADH is a finding noted during the evaluation process for other breast abnormalities.
      b. If ADH is diagnosed during needle biopsy, there are additional costs associated with surgical excision to rule out coexisting ductal carcinoma in situ (DCIS).

   3. *Risk reduction options.*
      a. Chemoprevention with tamoxifen reduces risk by 86%.[5]
      b. These individuals may elect to follow the increased surveillance recommendations suggested for women with Modified Gail Model Risk Assessment greater than 1.67% (Table 13.2).

C. Therapeutic radiation exposure

   1. *Exposure of breast to therapeutic radiation, such as mantle radiation of the chest wall, in women under age 30 may contribute to a 1% incidence of breast cancer per year beginning 10 years after treatment.[6]*

   2. *Cost associated with therapeutic radiation exposure is due to increased screening cost (Table 13.2 and Table 13.3). Data regarding cost effectiveness of intensive screening of this population is not reported.*

   3. *These individuals may elect to follow the increased surveillance recommendations suggested for women with therapeutic radiation exposure (Table 13.2)*

V. **Breast Cancer Screening for BRCA1 and BRCA2**

   A. Recommendations prior to age 25

   1. *Annual physical exams are encouraged by the National Comprehensive Cancer Network (NCCN).[7] Breast self-exams are also encouraged. This recommendation adds no additional cost to routine screening when compared to the most conservative recommendation for women under age 40 who are at no increased risk for breast cancer. Physical exams are encouraged every 1 to 3 years for average risk. In BRCA-positive women, there may be increased costs due to evaluation of patients' palpable concerns found on breast self-exam (see breast self-exam).*

   B. Recommendations at age 25 or older (Table 13.2)

   1. *Annual mammograms or mammograms beginning 5 to 10 years prior to the age of the youngest relative at diagnosis are*

TABLE 13.3 Cost of Additional Screening for Individuals at Increased Risk of Breast or Ovarian Cancer

Recommended Screening	Interval in Women of Average Risk	Interval in Women at High Risk	Additional Number of Exams/Tests in High-Risk Women	Estimated Costs per Test/Exam (conservative)	Estimated Costs per Test/Exam (upper range)	Additional Lifetime Cost for Intensive Screening
Physical Exam	Every 1–3 years age 20 to 39; Annually age 40 to 70	Every 6 months age 25 to 70	45	$98	$196	$4,410 to $8,820
Mammogram	Annually age 40 to 70	Annually age 25 to 70	15	$106	$108	$1,590 to $1,612
Transvaginal Ultrasound	Not recommended for screening	Every 6 months age 30 to 70	80	$103	$438	$8,240 to $35,040
CA–125	Not recommended for screening	Every 6 months age 50* to 70	40	$15	$106	$600 to $4,240

*Serum levels may be elevated in premenopausal women. Many facilities, however, begin testing at an earlier age than 50.

Adapted from Levine A, Hughes KS. Cost effectiveness of the identification of women at high risk for the development of breast and ovarian cancer. In: Vogel VG, ed. *Management of Patients at High Risk for Breast Cancer.* Malden, MA: Blackwell Science, Inc; 2001;262–276.

suggested. The Cancer Genetics Study Consortium suggests that BRCA-positive women begin annual mammograms at the age of 25 to 35 years.[8] Assuming that mammograms begin at the age of 25 and continue annually until age 40 when mammograms would begin for the general population, this would add 15 additional mammograms to the cost of a woman's lifetime care. Based on personal correspondence with C. Crissey, the estimated cost for screening mammogram is approximately $106 to $108.[9]

2. Clinical breast exams (CBEs) are recommended on a 6-month basis starting at age 25. Assuming that women of average risk follow the most conservative screening interval of annual CBEs, this recommendation adds one additional exam each year between the ages of 25 and 70 for a total of 45 additional office visits to the cost of care. The cost of an office visit with a skilled clinician has been calculated in the range of $98[9] to $196, according to personal correspondence with Crissey.

3. MRI is currently used in research settings, but may have a future role in BRCA-positive women where routine screening methods appear to have a low sensitivity. Breast cancers may appear at a younger age in this population, and mammography is not well suited to the dense breast of young women.[10] The cost effectiveness of this imaging modality cannot be estimated at this time.

4. With additional exams and earlier breast imaging, there will be abnormal findings that require further evaluation. The rate of false-positive tests will vary with the expertise of the diagnostic imaging facility, but even with highly skilled radiologists, the false-positive rate may be significant when screening young women with dense breasts for breast cancer. A conservative estimate of a 33% in additional cost for evaluation of false-positive findings would add between $1,980[9] and $3,443 to the screening process (Table 13.4).

TABLE 13.4	Estimated Cost of Lifetime Breast Cancer Screening in Women with Genetic Predisposition or Family History of Breast Cancer at an Early Age	
Breast Cancer Screening	**Estimated Lifetime Cost (conservative)**	**Estimated Lifetime Cost (upper range)**
Physical Exam	$4,410	$8,820
Mammogram	$1,590	$1,612
Additional Testing for False Positive (total plus 33%)	$1,980 (33% of $6,000)	$3,443 (33% of $10,432)
Total	$7,980	$13,875

Adapted from Levine A, Hughes KS. Cost effectiveness of the identification of women at high risk for the development of breast and ovarian cancer. In: Vogel VG, ed. *Management of Patients at High Risk for Breast Cancer.* Malden, MA: Blackwell Science, Inc; 2001;262–276.

VI. Cost Effectiveness of Breast Screening Modalities
   A. Mammograms
      1. *The cost effectiveness of mammographic screening in women of average risk is age-dependent. Among women of average risk, there is controversy regarding the age to begin screening mammogram and the age to stop mammogram. There appears to be consensus that high-risk women need to begin screening at an earlier age.*
         a. Screening women of average risk between the ages of 50 and 69 appears to be cost effective in multiple studies. When a computer-generated model was used to predict cost effectiveness, women ages 50 to 69 screened with mammograms every other year had an increased life expectancy of 12 days and a reduction in breast cancer mortality of 27% when compared with women not screened. The cost per year of life saved due to mammogram performed once every two years between ages 50 and 69 was $21,400. To prevent one death, 270 women between the ages of 50 and 69 need to be screened.[11] While this interval is quoted in several studies, this does not reflect the current practice of annual mammograms in women over age 50.
         b. Mammographic screening in women of average risk age 40 to 49 significantly reduces the cost effectiveness of screening. When women age 40 to 49 were included in a computer model for cost effectiveness and calculated for screening mammograms every 18 months, life expectancy increased an additional 2.5 days and mortality was reduced an additional 16%. The cost per year of life saved increased from $21,400 (in the 50 plus screening) to $105,000. In addition, 2,500 women between ages 40 to 49 would need to be screened to prevent one death in this age group compared with 270 women in the 50 plus age group.[11]
         c. The cost effectiveness of screening women of average risk after age 69 is also controversial. Cost estimations have been made using a computer model to predict cost in three screening options in women over age 69. One option was to stop routine screening mammograms after age 69. A second option offered screening biennial mammograms until age 79 in all women except those with the lowest quartile bone mineral density test (BMD). Increased BMD is a marker for higher lifetime estrogen exposure and higher risk for breast cancer. The last option was to continue biennial mammograms in women until age 79. Screening only those women with higher BMD on a biannual basis between ages 70 and 79 would prevent 9.4 deaths and add 2.1 days of life expectancy. This screening pattern would cost $66,773 per year of life saved, compared to biennial mammogram screening of all women between ages 70 and 79, which would cost $117,689 per year of life saved. Screening all women in their seventies would prevent 1.4 deaths and would add only 7.2 hours to life expectancy.[12]
      2. *In women at high risk for breast cancer, annual screening mammograms are suggested at an earlier age than the general population. The efficacy of mammograms starting at an early age remains controversial.*
         a. Given the increased incidence of breast cancer in the moderate- to high-risk population, presumably fewer women would need to be screened to prevent one death.

b. Breast cancer also appears at earlier ages in high-risk women, particularly with BRCA-positive women, and mammograms may be beneficial at an earlier age in this population.

c. Mammographic evaluations of young women with dense breasts are difficult to interpret, however, and may require additional studies to clarify findings.

d. There are data to suggest that current screening guidelines may be insufficient in women identified to be at high risk of breast cancer. Almost 1,200 women with a significant family risk for breast cancer were followed in one study.

　i. Among 128 women who were BRCA1 and BRCA2 positive, five of the nine breast cancers detected during an average three years of surveillance were identified during screening exams.

　ii. The remaining four breast cancers found in the BRCA-positive women were interval cancers.

　iii. There were no interval cancers found in BRCA mutation-negative women with an estimated lifetime risk of breast cancer of 15 to 30%.

　iv. Breast cancers may have been missed in the BRCA mutation-positive group due to difficulty identifying early cancers with mammogram in women with dense breasts.

　v. The second explanation is that the breast cancers diagnosed in BRCA-positive women appeared to have higher proliferative rates, suggesting more rapid growth.

　vi. Sixty-two percent of women with breast cancer under the age of 40 and 56% of BRCA-positive women had lymph node involvement at the time of diagnosis when compared to the study average of 35%.[10]

e. More frequent screening or screening with alternative tools, such as MRI, may have a future role in this special population.

B. Clinical Breast Exam (CBE)

1. *CBE is recommended by the Cancer Genetics Studies Consortium every 6 or 12 months starting at age 25 to 35 years for BRCA-positive women based on expert opinion, but note that benefit is not proven.[8] This is also recommended in women with prior thoracic radiation, women with LCIS, and women with strong family histories of breast cancer.[7]*

2. *This intervention doubles the number of clinic visits and may increase the number of diagnostic procedures for benign palpable abnormalities. Clinical breast exams performed by skilled health care providers have been suggested to be effective at reducing breast cancer mortality in the Canadian National Breast Screening Study–2.[13]*

C. Breast Self-Exam (BSE)

1. *BSE, while widely recommended, has not been demonstrated to be cost effective in women of average risk. The cost to teach enough women to produce one competent self-examiner has been estimated to be between $574 and $848.[14]*

2. *The Canadian Task Force on Preventive Health Care[15] suggested that instruction of breast self-exam be excluded from periodic health assessment.*

a. There are no data that predict the cost effectiveness of BSE in women at increased risk for breast cancer; however, an increase in office visits to evaluate benign breast concerns and an increase in benign biopsy has been associated with breast self-exam in the general population.

    b. No difference was noted in deaths from breast cancer or in the stage when the cancer was detected in women performing BSE when compared to women who do not perform this exam. While instruction appears to increase the sensitivity of BSE, it also appears to increase the number of false-positive findings.[15]

    c. The U.S. Preventative Services Task Force has neither recommended for or against instruction in BSE. This recommendation is currently under review. The National Comprehensive Cancer Network does encourage monthly breast self-exams starting by age 20; however, this recommendation is optional as benefit has not been proven.[7]

D. Screening and Morbidity and Mortality

    1. *The intention of screening programs is to identify breast cancer at an earlier stage and reduce breast cancer mortality.*

    2. *Costs associated with the diagnosis and management of breast disease are difficult to assess. The Agency for Healthcare Research and Quality found that minimal research was done on this topic and that results were too disparate to draw conclusions on cost effectiveness of interventions.[4] Several studies have found that prior screening, patient age, and the breast cancer stage at diagnosis significantly affects cost of treatment.*

    a. In a study of newly diagnosed breast cancer patients, those women with screening mammograms were more likely to be diagnosed at an earlier stage than women not previously screened.[16] In addition, the screened population also had lower treatment costs in the first year after diagnosis than the unscreened population ($15,100 for the group previously screened, compared to $19,000 for women who did not participate in screening).

    b. The cost to treat breast cancer increased as the stage at diagnosis increased. Younger age at diagnosis also increased costs due to longer lifetime follow-up cost and treatment of recurrence. A Canadian study[17] found Stage 1 breast cancers cost $23,275 per woman's lifetime, while Stage 4 breast cancers cost $36,340 per woman's lifetime. These costs are calculated in 1995 Canadian dollars and would be considerably higher today in the United States. Similar studies of breast cancer treatment and follow-up in the United States have lifetime costs that range from $36,926 in 1994 to $50,448 in 1992.

    c. While the intangible cost related to the loss of a loved one and the loss of productivity, both inside and outside the home, cannot be estimated, the financial burden of caring for individuals dying of breast cancer is significant. Health care costs associated with terminal breast cancer have been calculated to be over $36,000 Canadian dollars.[18]

VII. **Ovarian Cancer Screening for Mutation Carriers**

A. Women who are positive for BRCA1 or BRCA2 have an estimated risk for ovarian cancer between 26 and 40% by age 70.

B. Screening for individuals at increased risk of ovarian cancer (Table 13.3).

1. *The Cancer Genetics Studies Consortium[8] recommendations include both transvaginal ultrasound and CA–125 blood tests and are suggested every 6 months to annually beginning at age 25 to 35.*

2. *The National Institutes of Health (NIH) suggests transvaginal ultrasound and CA–125 laboratory analysis be performed every 6 months to annually starting at age 35 for women with inherited risk of ovarian cancer.[19]*

3. *Transvaginal ultrasounds.*

   a. Transvaginal ultrasound is used in the evaluation for ovarian cancer but does not distinguish well between benign and malignant findings, particularly in ovulating women. Even when use of this test is limited to high-risk women, there is a high false-positive rate[8] which increases the cost of evaluation.

   b. Personal correspondence from R. Thompson indicates the estimated cost of transvaginal ultrasound ranges between $103[9] and $438. When performed twice per year beginning at age 30 and continuing to age 70, this would add 80 additional tests to the cost of care (Table 13.3 and Table 13.5).

4. *Serum CA–125.*

   a. Serum CA–125 levels are a nonspecific tumor marker for ovarian cancer. Elevated levels may predict asymptomatic ovarian cancer; however, less than 50% of early stage ovarian cancers produce high levels. In addition, multiple benign conditions may cause an elevation of this marker, including pregnancy, benign gynecologic conditions such as endometriosis and pelvic inflammatory disease, and nongynecologic malignancies. Use of this test as a screening tool in the average-risk woman is not recommended.[20]

   b. Transvaginal ultrasound may improve specificity of this test at an additional cost.[8]

TABLE 13.5	Lifetime Cost of Ovarian Cancer Screening in BRCA1-Positive Women or Women with Strong Family History of Ovarian Cancer	
Ovarian Cancer Screening	**Estimated Lifetime Cost (conservative)**	**Estimated Lifetime Cost (upper range)**
Transvaginal Ultrasound	$8,240	$35,040
CA–125	$600	$4,240
Additional Testing for False Positive (total plus 33%)	$2,917 (33% of $8,840)	$12,962 (33% of $39,280)
Total	$11,757	$52,242

Adapted from Levine A, Hughes KS. Cost effectiveness of the identification of women at high risk for the development of breast and ovarian cancer. In: Vogel VG, ed. *Management of Patients at High Risk for Breast Cancer.* Malden, MA: Blackwell Science, Inc; 2001;262–276.

    c. Estimated cost of serum CA–125 may vary widely depending on the facility (Table 13.3) with a range of $15[9] to $106, according to personal communication with Crissey.

    d. Since serum levels may be elevated due to benign causes in premenopausal women, semiannual screening may be delayed until menopause or age 50 in some facilities. Using this conservative scenario, 40 additional tests for CA–125 would be added to the cost of care[9] (Table 13.3 and Table 13.5).

  5. Screening for ovarian cancer may necessitate repeated short-term transvaginal ultrasounds and laproscopic surgeries. Assuming 33% in additional cost to evaluate false positives, this would add $2,917[9] to $12,962 to the cost of ovarian cancer screening (Table 13.5).

  6. There is no data to demonstrate that bimanual pelvic examination is either sensitive or specific enough to identify ovarian cancer at an early stage.[20]

VIII. **Controversies Regarding Screening High-Risk Population**

  A. The cost of increased surveillance must be balanced against the benefit of early detection. In general, an intervention that results in a cost of less than $50,000 per year of life saved is considered to be cost effective. This figure appears to be somewhat arbitrary and does not appear to be adjusted over time. If this figure of $50,000 were adjusted for inflation, several of the interventions reviewed here would be considered to be cost effective.

  B. Variability in costs of screening and treatment modalities can be expected depending on the setting where the service is provided. For example, a transvaginal ultrasound performed in an office setting may be slightly more than $100 versus a transvaginal ultrasound performed and interpreted by an ultrasonographer in a cancer center which would cost over $400 (Table 13.3). This variability in costs creates a lifetime cost to screen for breast cancer that ranges between $7,980 and $13,875. Lifetime costs to screen for both breast and ovarian cancer would range between $19,737, using conservative cost estimations, and $66,117 using the higher cost estimations (Table 13.6).

TABLE 3.6	Total Cost of Screening for Breast and Ovarian Cancer	
Lifetime Cost to Screen	**Conservative Estimation of Cost**	**Upper Range of Cost**
Breast Cancer	$7,980	$13,875
Breast and Ovarian Cancer	$19,737	$66,117

Adapted from Levine A, Hughes KS. Cost effectiveness of the identification of women at high risk for the development of breast and ovarian cancer. In: Vogel VG, ed. *Management of Patients at High Risk for Breast Cancer.* Malden, MA: Blackwell Science, Inc; 2001:262–276.

C. Current screening tools and schedules may not be effective in high-risk women. In a study of 63 BRCA-positive women who elected not to have prophylactic mastectomy, eight breast cancers were identified over three years of intensive screening. Of significance, four of the eight breast cancers were diagnosed between scheduled 6-month clinical exams. Four of the eight breast cancers presented as palpable masses, and two cases had spread to lymph nodes by the time of diagnosis, suggesting either rapid growth or failure to identify the cancer at an earlier stage.[21]

IX. Prevention

A. Prophylactic mastectomy

1. *Mastectomy may be an acceptable risk reduction option for very high-risk individuals, including BRCA1- or BRCA2-positive women. Prophylactic mastectomy appears to reduce the incidence of breast cancer by approximately 90% in both high-risk women and moderate-risk women. More significantly, bilateral prophylactic mastectomies appear to reduce the risk of death related to breast cancer by 81 to 94%.[22]*

2. *Bilateral prophylactic mastectomy is a costly procedure, with or without reconstruction, but is considered a cost-effective procedure when an appropriate population is correctly targeted (Table 13.7).[3]*

3. *There are multiple intangible costs such as disruption of body image and altered perception of sexuality associated with mastectomy. Prior to undergoing such a procedure, the risks versus the benefits of this procedure must be clarified for the patient. Counseling that includes correct assessment of breast cancer risk is essential and would add to the cost of the procedure. Genetic testing may also be appropriate. In addition, women must understand that this procedure reduces but does not eliminate breast cancer risk.*

TABLE 13.7	Cost Effectiveness of Prophylactic Surgeries in Women of Ashkenazi Descent			
Treatment	Treatment at Age 30		Treatment at Age 40	
	Survival (days)	Cost per Year of Life Saved	Survival (days)	Cost per Year of Life Saved
Mastectomy & Oophorectomy	38	$20,717	26	$40,626
Mastectomy	33	$29,970	19	$61,509
Oophorectomy	11	$72,780	10	$85,987
Surveillance	6	$134,273	No benefit	No benefit

From Grann VR, Whang W, Jacobson JS, et al. Benefits and costs of screening Ashkenazi Jewish women for BRCA1 and BRCA2. *J Clin Oncol* 1999;17:494–500.

B. Prophylactic oophorectomy

1. Bilateral prophylactic oophorectomy appears to reduce ovarian cancer risk in high-risk women. The NIH recommends prophylactic oophorectomy at age 35 or at the completion of childbearing for women with an inherited risk for ovarian cancer.[19] This would include women with two first-degree relatives with ovarian cancer.

2. While the Cancer Genetic Studies Consortium fails to find sufficient evidence to recommend for or against the procedure for ovarian cancer risk reduction, they do suggest that BRCA1-positive women be offered prophylactic oophorectomy at age 35 or at the completion of childbearing.[8] In addition to ovarian cancer risk reduction, bilateral oophorectomy without mastectomy may confer a reduced risk for breast cancer in BRCA1-positive women.[23]

3. The efficacy of oophorectomy remains controversial. Many studies use a figure of 45% risk reduction. Screening asymptomatic women after oophorectomy would appear to have little benefit, and this would create cost savings when compared to intensive screening.

4. In addition to the cost of surgery, management of significant side effects may increase the long-term cost of this procedure. In the young women with functional ovaries, premature menopause from oophorectomy may require nonhormonal treatment of hot flashes, vaginal dryness, sleep disturbances, and osteoporosis risk. These would increase the cost of treatment by an unknown amount.

C. Combined prophylactic mastectomy and oophorectomy

1. Among women of Ashkenazi Jewish descent, genetic testing coupled with prophylactic surgeries may be cost effective in reducing cancer risks. Cost per year of life saved for a hypothetical population of women of Ashkenazi Jewish descent has been calculated. If all women in this population who tested positive for BRCA1 or BRCA2 elected to have prophylactic surgery at age 30, both mastectomy and combined mastectomy and oophorectomy would be cost effective. Oophorectomy alone, however, would not be cost effective using the $50,000 per year of life saved benchmark (Table 13.7).[3]

D. Chemoprevention (see also Chapter 7)

1. Tamoxifen reduced the risk of invasive breast cancer by 49% in the Breast Cancer Prevention Trial.[5] Risk reduction was greater in women with LCIS (56%) and atypical hyperplasia (86%). Estrogen receptor-positive cancers were reduced by 69% while estrogen negative cancers were not reduced. Tamoxifen also demonstrated a reduced risk of bone fractures but increased the risk of endometrial cancers and thromboembolic events.

   a. Tamoxifen may be cost effective when initiated in a woman in her early forties. When the savings from breast cancers prevented and hip fractures averted were balanced against treatment of side effects, including endometrial cancer and stroke, the cost to avoid a breast cancer in one woman would total $292,523. Assuming that tamoxifen was 100% effective and that all women with breast cancer would die of the disease, a woman in her forties would add 34.5 years to her life at a cost of $8,479 per year of life saved. However, the BCPT trial found tamoxifen to be effective at reducing breast cancers by approximately 50%, and this would increase the cost per year of life saved to $16,958. This is within the $50,000 per year of life saved ceiling generally used to estimate cost effectiveness if all women were expected to die from the disease. The cost per year of life saved would be significantly lower in women with LCIS (tamoxifen reduced risk by 56%) and with atypical hyperplasia (tamoxifen reduced risk by 86%).[24]

b. Using a computer model and survival data from Surveillance, Epidemiology, and End-Results (SEER), a much higher cost per year of life saved has been calculated with tamoxifen use. As the age of drug initiation increases, cost effectiveness decreases. The cost per year of life saved using this model has been calculated to be $46,619 when tamoxifen was initiated at age 35 in a hypothetical population of women with risk similar to the BCPT population. When tamoxifen was initiated after the age of 50, the threshold of $50,000 per year of life saved was exceeded.[25]

c. Similar costs per year of life saved have been calculated in other studies. High-risk women between ages 35 and 49 with LCIS or a 5-year risk of breast cancer equal to a 60-year-old woman were calculated to cost $41,372 per year of life saved. Women starting tamoxifen in their sixties would incur an estimated cost of $74,981 per year of life saved.[26]

d. Chemoprevention with tamoxifen may be cost effective in BRCA2 mutation-positive women but not BRCA1 mutation-positive women. Among participants in the National Surgical Adjuvant Breast and Bowel Project (NSABBP) Breast Cancer Prevention Trial (BCPT) there were 11 breast cancers in women positive for BRCA2 mutations. Eight of the 11 BRCA2 mutation-positive women who developed breast cancer were randomized to placebo, while three were randomized to tamoxifen. Tamoxifen appeared to reduce the risk for breast cancer by 62% in BRCA2-positive women, giving it a similar effectiveness as the general population. It should be noted that approximately 80% of the breast cancers in BRCA1-positive women are estrogen receptor (ER)-negative, and tamoxifen appears to reduce the risk of ER-positive breast cancers only. No risk reduction was seen in the BCPT for women with BRCA1.[27]

e. Women may overestimate their level of risk, and this creates a demand for medication to reduce breast cancer risk. A telephone survey of 1,273 women found 23% expressed an interest in using drug therapy for breast cancer prevention. In this study population, however, only 8% of the women were calculated to be at increased risk for breast cancer. Chemoprevention counseling is time intensive and primary care physicians may need assistance in counseling these women about breast cancer risk and chemoprevention.[28] Nurse practitioners may have a role in counseling and could lower the costs.

f. Other factors may influence cost effectiveness of tamoxifen.

   i. The cost of treatment has been calculated based on savings from breast cancers averted and reduced hip fractures. However, increased costs came from additional pap smears, evaluation for and treatment of endometrial cancer, strokes, transient ischemic attacks, pulmonary emboli, and deep vein thrombosis.[24] The clinician should certainly evaluate complaints of abnormal vaginal bleeding promptly in women using tamoxifen therapy. Women previously treated with hysterectomy have a lower cost per year of life saved, estimated at $46,060 per year of life saved compared to $74,981 per year of life saved for women started on tamoxifen in their sixties.[26]

    ii. Treatment and counseling due to increased menopausal symptoms with tamoxifen therapy may add additional costs. Women who have previously used hormone replacement may benefit from a period of no treatment prior to initiating tamoxifen so that baseline menopausal symptoms as well as patient tolerance to the symptoms can be assessed.

    iii. The cost of the drug adds to the cost of treatment. Most studies use a cost of $3,500 over five years for the drug.

2. *STAR (Study of Tamoxifen and Raloxifene) Trial.*

    a. Individuals who are postmenopausal and at increased risk for breast cancer may be considered for participation in the STAR Trial. This is a multicenter, double-blind study with no placebo group. Participants receive active drug for five years.

    b. The cost associated with the study would include routine screening and travel to the study site every 6 months for a total of 7 years (5 years of active treatment and 2 years of follow-up).

3. *Combined Oral Contraceptives (COCs).*

    a. The use of combined oral contraceptives (COCs) reduces the risk for ovarian cancer by approximately 30 to 34% in women of average risk who have ever used COCs, and reduces risk by 45 to 70% in those women who have used COCs for more than six years. Women positive for BRCA1 or BRCA2 have a similar reduction with COC use, decreasing risk for ovarian cancer by 20% with up to three years of use and by 60% with six or more years of use.[29]

    b. These drugs are generally low cost and well tolerated. COCs provide multiple nontangible benefits, including highly effective contraception and reduction of menstrual irregularities.

    c. Correct selection of appropriate candidates for use of oral contraceptives as well as for patient satisfaction requires counseling and follow-up to evaluate for symptoms.

X. Cost Effectiveness of Specialty Resource Facility/Clinic

    A. A specialty cancer screening and prevention clinic may be the most effective resource for managing women at increased risk for breast cancer. The issues outlined previously are complex and require extensive time and expertise to direct women through appropriate options. Those women of average risk need to be identified and returned to less costly cancer screening.

    B. A multidisciplinary team is required to provide a correct balance of knowledge and cost effectiveness.

        1. *Midlevel providers with special knowledge may function well in multiple areas.*

      a. Genetic risk assessment counselor

      b. General risk assessment and prevention counseling

      c. Clinical exams and breast cancer screening

2. *Specialists within the clinic or ready referral sources are essential.*

      a. The screening guidelines outlined previously rely extensively on diagnostic imaging. Radiologists with expertise in breast screening are crucial to the prompt identification of potentially subtle changes in the breasts. Ideally, a diagnostic imaging clinic located on-site expedites the evaluation of suspicious findings.

      b. An on-site surgical specialty clinic or local referral sources that include plastic surgeons and breast surgical oncologists can facilitate treatment of suspicious findings.

      c. Medical breast oncologists and gynecology oncologists will also be essential for the care of high-risk women.

C. By moving the screening of the moderate- to high-risk population out of PCP's office and into a specialty clinic, a more cost-effective use of resources can be realized. The primary care provider is freed from extensive counseling and follow-up of a high-risk population. Women may have their risk assessed more accurately, and those found to be of average risk may be returned to routine follow-up, reducing unnecessary screening.

D. The specialty clinic acts as a research center for chemoprevention trials such as STAR and possibly research trials on imaging techniques, such as MRI.

E. There are liability issues surrounding breast cancer. Failure to diagnose or delay in diagnosis of breast cancer is the most common cause of malpractice litigation.[4]

1. *Intensive screening of high-risk individuals is considered the standard of care.*

2. *Failure to warn women unaware of their level of risk of screening or risk reduction options may be a medical/legal liability. Health care providers have a responsibility to recognize individuals at increased risk and then have a duty to warn them of this risk without being asked. Patients also require sufficient information to make an informed decision regarding testing and risk reduction strategies. Understanding of risks and benefits is especially important for individuals considering genetic testing.[30,31]*

XI. Conclusion

A. The effectiveness of various screening and cancer prevention interventions remains controversial, particularly among women considered to be at increased risk for both breast and ovarian cancer. Screening recommendations for women at average risk of breast cancer may be inadequate for women at high risk. There is a lack of data to support the effectiveness of some interventions currently recommended, such as breast self-exam, and a lack of data to support an appropriate interval for screening.

B. The cost of both screening and prevention modalities varies widely. Cost effectiveness is difficult to assess due to lack of studies or lack of standardization between studies. Mammographic recommendations and cost are an example of this problem with studies performed worldwide using different recommendations with wide variations in fee structure.

C. Many procedures fall outside of traditional cost effectiveness. The use of $50,000 as the benchmark for cost effectiveness may need to be rethought and adjusted to reflect the current cost of living.

D. Issues surrounding breast cancer risk and risk reduction are complex and controversial. Counseling women regarding their risks appears to be essential to developing a plan of care that is effective and acceptable to both the provider and patient. This is a niche that can be filled by the midlevel provider; however, reimbursement issues may limit access to this essential service.

References

1. Mundinger MA, Kane RL, Lenz ER, et al. Primary care outcomes in patients treated by nurse practitioners or physicians: a randomized trial. *JAMA* 2000;283:59–69.

2. Venning P, Durie A, Roland M, et al. Randomised controlled trial comparing cost effectiveness of general practitioners and nurse practitioners in primary care. *BMJ* 2000;320:1048–1053.

3. Grann VR, Whang W, Jacobson JS, et al. Benefits and costs of screening Ashkenazi Jewish women for BRCA1 and BRCA2. *J Clin Oncol* 1999;17:494–500.

4. *Diagnosis and management of specific breast abnormalities. Summary, evidence report/technology assessment: Number 33.* Rockville, MD: Agency for Healthcare Research and Quality; April 2001. AHRQ publication 01-E045. Available at: *http://www.ahrq.gov/clinic/abnorsum.htm.*

5. Fisher B, Costantino JP, Wickerham DL, et al. Tamoxifen for prevention of breast cancer: report of the National Surgical Adjuvant Breast and Bowel Project P–1 Study. *J Natl Cancer Inst* 1998;90:1371–1388.

6. Goss PE, Sierra S. Current perspectives on radiation-induced breast cancer. *J Clin Oncol* 1998;16:338–347.

7. NCCN Breast Cancer Screening Guidelines. *The Complete Library of NCCN Oncology Practice Guidelines* [book on CD-ROM]. Rockledge, PA: National Comprehensive Cancer Network;2001. To view the most recent version of the guideline, see *www.nccn.org.*

8. Burke W, Daly M, Garber J, et al. Recommendations for follow-up care of individuals with inherited predisposition to cancer: II. BRCA1 and BRCA2. *JAMA* 1997;277:997–1003.

9. Levine A, Hughes KS. Cost effectiveness of the identification of women at high risk for the development of breast and ovarian cancer. In: Vogel VG, ed. *Management of Patients at High Risk for Breast Cancer.* Malden, MA: Blackwell Science, Inc; 2001:262–276.

10. Brekelmans CTM, Seynaeve C, Bartels CCM, et al. Effectiveness of breast cancer surveillance in BRCA1/2 gene mutation carriers and women with high familial risk. *J Clin Oncol* 2001;19:924–930.

11. Salzmann P, Kerlikowske K, Phillips K. Cost effectiveness of extending screening mammography guidelines to include women 40 to 49 years of age. *Ann Intern Med* 1997;127:955–965.

12. Kerlikowske K, Salzmann P, Phillips KA, et al. Continuing screening mammography in women aged 70 to 79 years: impact on life expectancy and cost-effectiveness. *JAMA* 1999;282:2156–2163.

13. Miller AB, To T, Baines CJ, Wall C. Canadian National Breast Screening Study–2: 13-year results of a randomized trial in women aged 50–59 years. *J Natl Cancer Inst* 2000;92:1490–1499.

14. O'Malley M. Cost effectiveness of two nurse-led programs to teach breast self-examination. *Am J Prev Med* 1993;9:139–145.

15. Baxter N. Preventive health care, 2001 update: Should women be routinely taught breast self-examination to screen for breast cancer? *CMAJ* 2001;164:1837–1846.

16. Legorreta AP, Brooks RJ, Leibowitz AN, Solin LJ. Cost of breast cancer treatment: a 4-year longitudinal study. *Arch Intern Med* 1996;156:2197–2201.

17. Will BP, Berthelot JM, Le Petit C, et al. Estimates of the lifetime costs of breast cancer treatment in Canada. *Eur J Cancer* 2000;36:724–735.

18. Wai ES, Trevisan CH, Taylor SC, et al. Health system costs of metastatic breast cancer. *Breast Cancer Res Treatment* 2001;65:233–240.

19. NIH Consensus Development Panel on Ovarian Cancer. NIH Consensus Conference: Ovarian cancer-screening, treatment and follow-up. *JAMA* 1995;273:491–497.

20. National Cancer. *Genetics of breast and ovarian cancer (PDQ). Cancer genetics— health professionals.* [Cancer Net Web site] Available at: http://cancernet.nci.nih.gov. Accessed August 2001.

21. Meijers-Heijboer H, van Geel B, van Putten WLJ, et al. Breast cancer after prophylactic bilateral mastectomy in women with BRCA1 or BRCA2 mutation. *N Engl J Med* 2001;345:159–164.

22. Hartmann LC, Sellers TA, Schaid DJ, et al. Efficacy of bilateral prophylactic mastectomies in BRCA1 and BRCA2 gene mutation carriers. *J Natl Cancer Inst* 2001;93:1633–1637.

23. Rebbeck TR, Levin AM, Eisen A, et al. Breast cancer risk after bilateral oophorectomy in BRCA1 mutation carriers. *J Natl Cancer Inst* 1999;91:1475–1479.

24. Smith TJ, Hillner BE. Tamoxifen should be cost-effective in reducing breast cancer risk in high-risk women. *J Clin Oncol* 2000;18:284–286.

25. Grann VR, Sundararajan V, Jacobson JS, et al. Decision analysis of tamoxifen for the prevention of invasive breast cancer. *Cancer J from Sci Am* 2000;6:169–178.

26. Noe LL, Becker RV 3rd, Gradishar WJ, et al. The cost effectiveness of tamoxifen in the prevention of breast cancer. *Am J Managed Care* 1999;5(suppl 6): S389–S406.

27. King MC, Weiand S, Hale K, et al. Tamoxifen and breast cancer incidence among women with inherited mutations in BRCA1 and BRCA2. *JAMA* 2001;286:2251–2256.

28. Bastian LA, Lipkus IM, Kuchibhafla MN, et al. Women's interest in chemoprevention for breast cancer. *Arch Intern Med* 2001;161:1639–1644.

29. Narod SA, Risch H, Moslehi R, et al. Oral contraceptives and the risk of hereditary ovarian cancer. *N Engl J Med* 1998;339:424–428.

30. Dickens BM, Pei N, Taylor K. Legal and ethical issues in genetic testing and counselling for susceptibility to breast, ovarian and colon cancer. *Can Med Assoc J* 1996;154:813–818.

31. Macdonald KG, Doan B, Kelner M, Taylor KM. A sociobehavioural perspective on genetic testing and counselling for heritable breast, ovarian and colon cancer. *Can Med Assoc J* 1996;154:457–464.

A